JN065040

杉山和一が創案した「十四管術」の実践

日本鍼灸の極意

管鍼法
かんしんほう

北川 毅・著
大浦 慈観・監修
マクギバン美登利・英語共著

【日英対訳版】
Japanese
&
English
Bilingual Book

BAB JAPAN

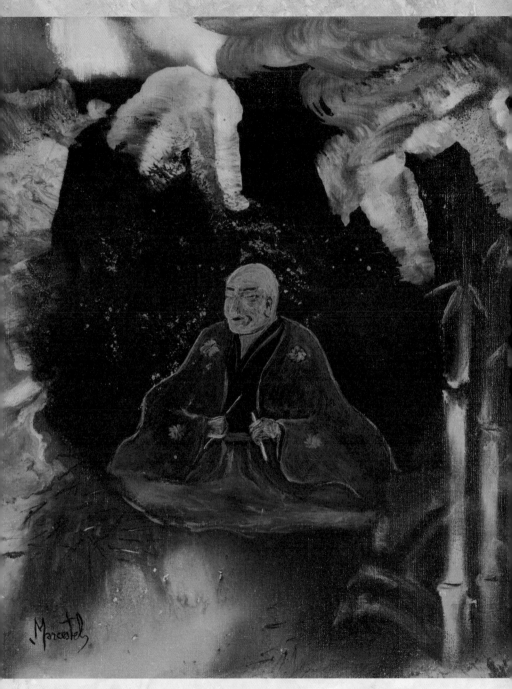

杉山和一・肖像画（マーク・エステル作）

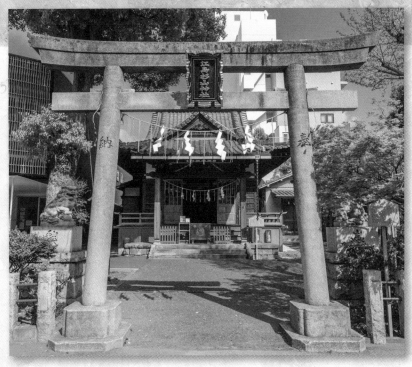

江島杉山神社（東京都墨田区）

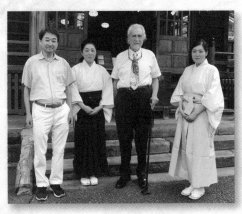

2021年8月、マーク・エステル氏が杉山和一の肖像画（前頁）を江島杉山神社に奉納した（左より、著者、田部裕子宮司、マーク・エステル氏、田部景子権禰宜）

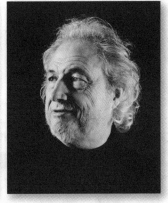

フランス人アーティスト、マーク・エステル氏。伊勢神宮をはじめとする全国180社以上の神社に、日本神話を題材とした作品を奉納。2014年「文化関係者文部科学大臣表彰」受賞

2010年頃より、海外で鍼灸の臨床と教育活動に携わる機会が増え、その業務経験を通じて、私は「日本鍼灸」ということを強く意識するようになりました。私が外国人から最も多く尋ねられる質問は、「日本の鍼灸と中国の針灸の違いは何か?」ということです。同時に、外国人の専門家の多くが、「針が細い」「鍼管を使って針を打つ」ということが日本の鍼灸の特徴であると認識しています。

針灸は、6世紀に中国から日本に伝来し、日本では独自の変容を遂げていきました。そして、その起点となったのが、17世紀の杉山和一（すぎやまわいち）による「鍼管」の創案と「管鍼法」の確立です。現在では、刺針法としての管鍼法は、日本国内のみならず、世界の刺針法の標準となりつつあり、杉山和一の名は、海外の専門家の間で "The father of Japanese acupuncture"（日本の鍼の父）として専門家の尊敬の念を集めています。

このように、管鍼法や細い針がグローバル化している現状において、私たち日本人鍼灸師は、「日本の鍼灸と中国の針灸の違いは何か?」という海外の専門家の疑問に対して、明確に答えられなくてはなりません。

そして、そのためには、管鍼法とその創案者である杉山和一について、一定の知識を身に付けておくことが必要となりますが、現状では、鍼灸師の養成施設で使用されている教科書の管鍼法と杉山和一に関する記載は決して十分であるとは言えません。そこで、私たちは本書を執筆しました。

このような事情をご理解くださり、日英対訳という形で本書の出版の機会を与えてくださいましたBABジャパンの東口敏郎社長と編集担当の森口敦氏に厚く御礼申し上げます。そして、杉山和一研

究の第一人者であり本書の監修を務めてくださいました大浦慈観先生、約1年間にわたり、英語の原稿を一緒に書いてくださったマクギバン美登利先生、実技の写真撮影にご協力いただいた加納覚先生、本書の出版に全面的にご協力くださった江島杉山神社の田部裕子宮司様、田部景子権禰宜様に厚く御礼申し上げます。

本書の著者は私ですが、立場、持ち場がそれぞれに異なる日本人鍼灸師がチームを組み、一丸となって完成させた日本鍼灸に関する書籍であり、このチームは私の誇りです。

本書の執筆中に、フランス人アーティストで、日本神話の作家であるマーク・エステル氏が、脳梗塞を発症して利き手側の右半身に麻痺が残りましたが、懸命なリハビリと鍼灸治療によって再び作品を制作できるまでに回復しました。そこで、彼は杉山和一を作品に描き、江島杉山神社に奉納されました。

この時期に、日本神話の世界を描き続けてきた作家が鍼灸によって健康を回復し、鍼灸の神様が御祭神として祀られる神社に作品を奉納したというのは、何とも奇遇な出来事ですので、その作品を口絵でご紹介させていただきました。ぜひ、江島杉山神社に足をお運びいただき、実物の作品をご覧ください。

著者　北川　毅

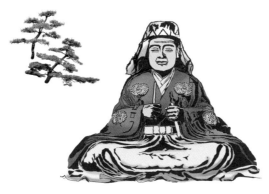

イラスト提供：江島杉山神社

CONTENTS

杉山和一・肖像画……2

はじめに……4

Chapter

1

管鍼法とは

◆ 管鍼法と管鍼術

◆ 管鍼法の英語表記について

9

Chapter

2

世界に広がる日本鍼灸

◆ Shinkyu とは

◆ Shinkyu の独自性

◆ Shinkyu の特徴と優位性

◆ 細い鍼灸針と管鍼法

◆ 丁寧で繊細

◆ 日本と日本人に対する信頼性

◆ 衛生的

◆ 洗練性

13

Chapter

3

鍼術と気

◆ 気を診て、気を操る

◆ 気に対する鍼術の作用

29

Chapter 4 刺針法としての管鍼法

◆ 世界標準の刺針法へ
◆ 鍼管
◆ 刺手と押手
◆ 挿管
◆ 切皮・弾入

39

Chapter 5 十四管術の実践

◆ 十四管術の目的と分類
◆ ① 針とともに叩く術
　細指管 Fine Finger Kan ／暁の管 Rising sun Kan ／気拍管 Ki-tapping Kan
◆ ② 針とともに推す術
　推指管 Finger pressing Kan ／爻綖管 Tube pressing Kan
◆ ③ 針の周囲を叩く、摩擦する術
　扣管 Tapping around Kan ／撥指管 Spring finger Kan ／遠覚管 Far sense Kan
◆ ④ 針を振動させる術
　随肉管 Muscle rubbing Kan
　竜頭管 Dragon's Head Kan ／巧指管 Ingenious Dragon's Head Kan
　爅鍼管 Glowing Needle Kan ／内調管 Internal tuning Kan
　通谷管 Connecting valley Kan

49

Chapter 6

管鍼法の創案者・杉山和一

◆ 日本鍼灸の父
◆ 盲目となり鍼医を志す
◆ 挫折を経て御神託を授かる
◆ 京で「管鍼法」を確立する
◆ 鍼術の教科書を編纂
◆ 徳川綱吉の侍医となり、『杉山真伝流』が完成

91

Chapter 7

杉山和一を祀る江島杉山神社

◆ 江戸の一大名所となる
◆ 江島杉山神社の境内
◆ 杉山和一と江島杉山神社にまつわる神々
◆ 江島杉山神社の特徴

107

Chapter 8

管鍼術の原点・江島神社（藤沢市）

◆ 杉山和一が御神託を得た神社
◆ 杉山和一木座像と生誕410年記念像

127

おわりに……132

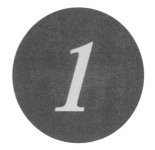

Chapter 1

管鍼法とは

◆ 管鍼法と管鍼術

「管鍼法」とは、「鍼管」と呼ばれる管を用いた鍼術における独自の技法であり、17世紀に、「杉山流」を創成した鍼医である杉山和一によって確立され、広められました。

杉山流は、和一の没後、二代目・三島安一の時代になって、関東から日本全国に広まっていきました。そして、三代目・島浦和田一は、杉山和一と三島安一の下で、杉山流の鍼治技術を理論化、体系化し、『杉山真伝流』という流儀書を完成させました。

管鍼法は、日本国外では一般に、「鍼管を用いた刺針法」として認識されています。しかし、杉山流では、鍼管は刺針だけを目的として用いられていたのではなく、刺針の効果を高めるための付加的な刺激を与えることにも用いられていました。

そして、そのために考案された数々の技法は「管鍼術」と呼ばれています。『杉山真伝流』には、十四種類の管鍼術が記載されており、それらの術は「十四管術」と名付けられています。

したがって、管鍼法は単なる刺針法ではなく、管鍼術を含めた「鍼管を用いた鍼術の技法全般」として正しく認識されることが必要です。

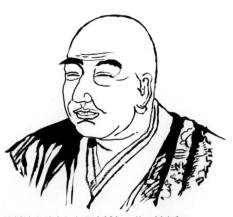

管鍼法を確立した日本鍼灸の父、杉山和一

10

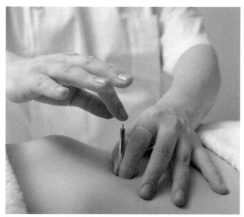
鍼管を用いた刺針法「管鍼法」

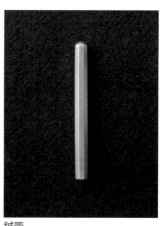
鍼管

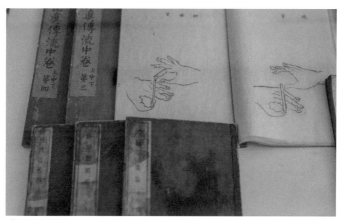
『杉山真伝流』

　また、「鍼管を用いた刺針法」、すなわち狭義の刺針法としての管鍼法は、狭義の管鍼法として位置付けられます。現在、日本の鍼灸師のほとんどが、この管鍼法を用いて刺針を行っており、管鍼法は、日本の標準的な刺針法となっています。

　そして、刺針法としての管鍼法は、この数年で海外諸国においても急速に普及し、刺針法の世界標準となりつつあります。

　このような世界的な現状から本書では、管鍼法を刺針法と管鍼術に分類し、国内外の専門家に向けて、管鍼法全般について詳しく解説していきます。

◆管鍼法の英語表記について

管鍼法は、英語の表記では広義においても狭義においても Kanshin Method という言葉が用いられます。そして、刺針法としての管鍼法を、広義の管鍼法と区別したい場合には、Kanshin Needling Method が用いられます。

一方、管鍼術は日本語の専門用語が英語としても採用されて Kanshin-Jutsu と表記されます。「術」とは、単なる「技術」ではなく、「技術」と「芸術」を合わせ持つ高水準の技術を意味する言葉であり、英語にはこれに該当する言葉が存在しません。そのため、英語圏においても、「術」という言葉が採用されて Jutsu と表記されます。

管鍼法（広義）/ 鍼管を用いた鍼術の技法全般
Kanshin Method

管鍼法（狭義）/ 鍼管を用いた刺針法
Kanshin Method / Kanshin Needling Method

管鍼術 / 鍼管を用いた副刺激術全般
Kanshin-Jutsu

十四管術 / 十四通りの管鍼術
Fourteen Kan Jutsu / Fourteen Kanshin-Jutsu

Chapter 2

世界に広がる日本鍼灸

◆ Shinkyu とは

管鍼法について正しく認識するためには、前提として、管鍼法を生み出した日本の鍼灸（Shinkyu）について、正しく知ることが重要です。そこで、本書では、最初に日本の鍼灸について解説します。

Shinkyu とは、日本語で「鍼」（acupuncture）と「灸」（moxibustion）という意味です。鍼と灸はそれぞれ異なる治療法ですが、多くの共通点があります。例えば、ともに東洋の伝統医学の治療法として、古くから実践されてきたこと、体表から人体に対して刺激を与える治療法であること、経穴と呼ばれる特有の治療点が用いられることなど、歴史、理論、手法などです。

そのため、東アジア諸国では、鍼と灸は、一体の治療法として実践され、日本では「鍼灸」と呼ばれてきました。

一方、ヨーロッパやアメリカなどの国々では、「acupuncture」という言葉は、広く認知されていますが、「灸」（moxibustion）や「艾」（moxa）は一般的な言葉として認知されていません。それらの国々では、鍼だけが単独で普及を遂げ、灸に対する認知度が低いことが理由でしょう。

鍼と灸には、それぞれ異なる効果と利点があります。そのため、患者さんの状態や訴えに基づき、必要に応じて鍼と灸のいずれか、もしくは両方が臨機応変に用いられるのが本来の姿です。また、両者を併用することで相乗効果が期待できる場合もあります。

そのため、鍼だけが単独で普及し、灸が置き去りにされているヨーロッパやアメリカの現状は、日本の専門家にとっては大きな違和感を感じるものです。東アジア以外の諸外国においても、鍼と灸は、鍼灸という一体の治療法として再認識されるべきであろうというのが私たちの見解です。

本書では、日本の鍼灸の独自性と優位性についてご理解いただくことを目的として、日本の鍼術の大きな特徴である管鍼法についてご紹介します。そのため、本書においては日本の鍼灸のうちの鍼術について解説していきますが、鍼と灸は、元来、「鍼灸」という一体の治療法であるということをご理解ください。

そして、日本由来の鍼灸（Japanese acupuncture & moxibustion）は「鍼灸」（Shinkyu）としてご認識いただきたいと思います。

私たちが日本で実践する鍼灸は日本独自のShinkyuであり、ヨーロッパやアメリカなどで単独で認知されているacupunctureとは異なるものです。そのため、本書をお読みくださる海外の専門家の皆様には、ぜひ"Shinkyu"という言葉と「鍼灸」という日本語の文字を覚えていただき、鍼と灸を一体の治療法として認識していただければ幸いです。

そして、できれば"Harikyu""Hari""Kyu""Okyu"という言葉も覚えていただきたいと思います。

Shinkyuは、日本語の文字では「鍼灸」と表記されます。「鍼」はacupunctureという意味で、「灸」はmoxibustionという意味です。

Acupunctureを意味する「鍼」という字には、2通りの読み方があり、"Shin"と発音される場合と"Hari"と発音される場合があります。そのため、「鍼灸」は、アルファベット表記では、"Shinkyu"ばかりでなく"Harikyu"と表記される場合もありますが、意味に相違はありません。本書では、表記の統一をはかるために"Shinkyu"を採用します。

また、「鍼」という言葉と文字が単独で用いられる場合は、通常は"Hari"と発音され、単独でShinと発音

したり、アルファベットで表記されることはありません。

一方、moxibustion は、日本語では "Kyu"（灸）または "Okyu"（お灸）と言いますが、"Okyu" の "O" は丁寧を表す日本語の接頭語であり、moxibustion を表す日本語の名詞は "Kyu" です。そして、"Okyu" の方がより丁寧な言い方となります。また、このように、"Kyu" を丁寧に表現する言葉として、"Okyu" という言葉は使われますが、"Hari" に対して "Ohari" という言葉が使われることはありません。

鍼灸は、6世紀に中国から伝来した針灸が、その後の長い時間の中で、日本において独自の発展を遂げたものです。中国の針灸も日本の鍼灸も、その基礎理論や鍼と灸を用いて治療するという「本質」に相違はありません。

基本的で普遍的な部分においては、両者の間に違いはなく、その違いは各論的な部分における理論、技法、使用する道具などにあります。鍼灸が日本において発展する課程では、様々な技法や道具が創案され、独自の変容を遂げながら日本鍼灸として発展していきました。

Shinkyu	: acupuncture & moxibustion
Harikyu	: acupuncture & moxibustion
Hari	: acupuncture
Kyu	: moxibustion
Okyu	: moxibustion（丁寧語）

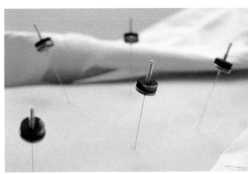

煙の出ない炭化艾

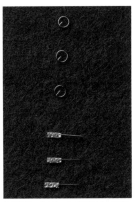

円皮針（上）と皮内針（下）

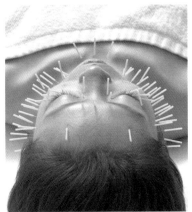

美容鍼灸

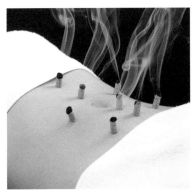

温筒灸

◆ **Shinkyu** の独自性

　日本において鍼灸が発展した過程では、管鍼法、細い針、ディスポーザブル鍼灸針などが創案され、日本鍼灸を象徴する独自の技法と道具として位置付けられています。

　他にも、日本では、置き針と呼ばれる円皮針や皮内針、温筒灸、煙の出ない炭化艾、美容を目的として鍼灸を用いる美容鍼灸など、多様な技術と道具が創案されています。そして、それらの技法や道具はいずれも、鍼灸の利用者が、より快適、安全、安心で効果の高い施術を受けられることを目標として、先人たちの絶え間ない努力によって創案されたものです。

◆ Shinkyu の特徴と優位性

　海外からの Shinkyu の施術や技術指導の依頼により、私はこれまでに数多くの国々を訪れてきました。そして、諸外国における業務経験を通じて、私は多くの人々が、Shinkyu に対して共通した印象や認識を持っていることを知りました。それは、Shinkyu に対する共通した一定の評価があるということであり、その評価は、日本の Shinkyu の特徴であることを示唆しています。

　そこで、私が諸外国における業務経験を通じて得てきた Shinkyu に対する評価について、整理してお話ししたいと思います。私自身が得てきた Shinkyu に対する評価は、主として次の通りです。

- ●細い鍼灸針と管鍼法
- ●丁寧で繊細
- ●日本と日本人に対する信頼性
- ●衛生的
- ●洗練性

◆ 細い鍼灸針と管鍼法

　17世紀において鍼灸は、日本では特に大きな変容を遂げました。そして、その最大の要因が、本書の題材で

ある「鍼管」と「管鍼法」です。

この時代、中国や日本の他の流派では、「撚針法（ねんしんほう）」という刺針法によって、太くて長い10番（直径0・34mm）～45番（直径1・04mm）程度の鉄と銀で作られた鍼灸針（以下：針）が使用されていました。

一方、杉山流では、「管鍼法」によって、推定で5番（直径0・24mm）～9番（直径0・32mm）の針が使用されていたとされています。そして、その後の針の製造技術の進歩により、既に19世紀には、日本では、02番（直径0・12mm）～1番（直径0・16mm）の極細針も使用されていました。

江戸時代に使われていた針と鍼管（所蔵：加納覚）

「撚針法」とは、母指と示指で針柄を持ち、針を捻りながら皮膚に対して直接刺入する刺針法です。この技法では、切皮の難易度が高く、刺針技術が未熟な場合には、針の刺入時に疼痛が生じる場合が少なくありません。

また、針の針体は、長ければ長いほど、また、細ければ細いほど、よりたわみやすくなる性質を持つことから、一定以上の太さの針でなければ、捻針法は用いることができません。

一方、鍼管を用いる管鍼法では、鍼管の内径が針体のたわみを防ぎ、鍼管の内径以上に針体がたわむことがないため、細い針であっても、針体を曲げることなく円滑に刺針を行うことができます。そのため、管鍼法の普及により、日本では、中国の針よりも大幅に細い針が使用されるようになりました。また、当時の日本の高度な針の製造技術は、細い針を作る上で

19

は不可欠な要素であったと言えるでしょう。

現代においても、臨床で一般的に使用される「針の太さ」が異なることは、日本鍼灸と中国針灸の大きな違いとして認められています。日本では、直径〇・一二〜〇・二六㎜の太さの針が一般的に使用されているのに対して、中国では直径〇・三〇㎜未満の針はおおよそ使用されていません。そのため、細い針を使用しているのが日本鍼灸であり、太い針を使用するのが中国針灸であると認識している専門家や利用者も少なくないようです。

日本における管鍼法と細い針の発明と普及は、鍼術の「革命」とも言える歴史的な出来事です。そして、日本独自の鍼灸は、管鍼法と細い針が誕生した一七世紀に開花し、そこを起点としてその歴史が始まりました。したがって、一七世紀は、日本鍼灸の歴史の原点であると言っても過言ではありません。

現在、日本には多様な流派の鍼灸が存在し、「標準」として認められている日本鍼灸の体系や手法は存在しません。したがって、日本において独自に発展を遂げた日本由来の鍼灸は、いずれも「日本鍼灸」として認めることができるでしょう。

一方、日本では、いずれの流派の鍼灸においても、管鍼法と極めて細い針が使用されることから、管鍼法と細い針は、日本鍼灸を象徴する技法と道具であり、日本鍼灸の大きな特徴として位置付けられてきました。そして、現在では、日本国内ばかりではなく、世界各地にも広く普及し、世界の鍼灸の標準的な手法と道具となりつつあります。

管鍼法と細い針は、いずれも鍼術の健全な普及と発展を願う杉山和一の熱意と努力によって生み出され、現代もなお、日本と世界の鍼術の世界に存在しているのです。そして、このような功績により、杉山和一は世界各地で「日本の鍼の父」（The father of Japanese acupuncture）と呼ばれています。

日本の針（上の 3 本）と中国の針（下の 5 本）〈実物大〉

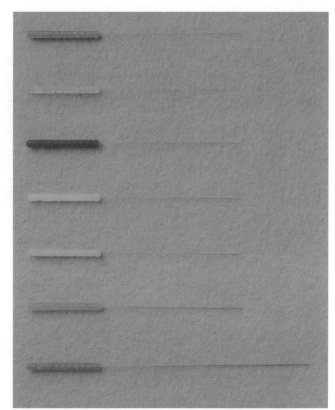

針の太さで針柄が色分けされたディスポーザブル鍼灸針〈実物大〉

日本では、針はその直径によって「号数」が定められており、針の太さは「直径」と「号数」によって明確化されています。そして、この号数は中国で使用されている号数とは異なるため、注意が必要です。

日本では、針の号数は、直径が0・02㎜増加するごとに号数の段階が増加し、10号針（直径0・10㎜）～50号針（直径0・50㎜）の21種類が規格化されています。

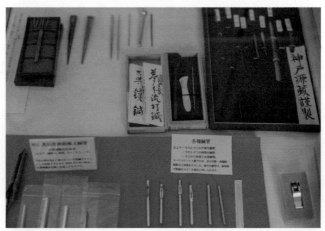

日本鍼灸の道具

針の太さの規格

直径	号数（日本）	番数（日本）	号数（中国）
0.12mm	12号	02 (00) 番	
0.14mm	14号	01番	
0.16mm	16号	1番	
0.18mm	18号	2番	
0.20mm	20号	3番	
0.22mm	22号	4番	35号
0.24mm	24号	5番	34号
0.26mm	26号	6番	33号
0.28mm	28号	7番	32号
0.30mm	30号	8番	31号
0.32mm	32号	9番	30号
0.34mm	34号	10番	29号
0.38mm	38号		28号
0.42mm	42号		27号
0.45mm	45号		26号

また、日本では、針の太さを表す単位として、規格化されている「号数」とは別の「番数」（番定）という単位も存在し、臨床現場や教育現場では「号数」よりも、むしろ「番数」の方が一般的に用いられています。針の番数は、直径が0・02㎜増加するごとに1番ずつ号数が増加し、日本では02番（直径0・12㎜）〜8番（直径0・30㎜）の針が、一般的に使用されています。

ディスポーザブル鍼灸針では、臨床現場で使用される針の太さの判別がつきやすくなるよう、太さによって針柄が色分けされているものもあります。

◆丁寧で繊細

諸外国の利用者の方々や専門家によるShinkyuに対する最も高い評価は、圧倒的に「丁寧」で「繊細」であるということです。鍼の施術は、他人の体に対して針を刺入するという侵襲行為を伴い、灸の施術には火を使うため、丁寧で繊細な施術を行うことは、極めて重要な要素となります。

そして、丁寧で繊細であるという理由から、昨今では、Shinkyu の技術を学びたがる専門家が世界各地で増えています。この数年、私は世界各地で美容鍼灸に関する講習会を積極的に開講してきましたが、受講者たちの受講動機は、単に美容鍼灸の技法を身に付けたいというばかりでなく、日本の Shinkyu についてもっと深く知りたいということも動機である場合が少なくありません。

◆日本と日本人に対する信頼性

海外に長く滞在して実感することは、"Japanese" "made in Japan" "from Japan" など、"Japan" "Japanese" とつくだけで、世界中のどこへ行っても、その製品やサービスは「安心」で「安全」であり、同時に「一流」であると認知されているということです。

例えば、家庭電化製品、自動車、時計などは、いずれも日本人が発明したものではありません。ところが、日本製のそれらの製品は世界を席巻し、"Made in Japan "という言葉は、日本と日本人による仕事そのものを、世界のブランドにしてしまいました。"Japan" と "Japanese" は、安定した信頼のブランドとして認められているのです。

そして、一つの国として、このような事例は、世界中でも他にはありません。このような現状から、日本由来の鍼灸は、"Shinkyu" という日本語を標榜するべきであろうというのが私たちの見解です。

24

◆衛生的

日本と日本人の印象を表す言葉として、"clean"（清潔）ということがよく言われます。日本を訪れた外国人の中には、トイレの清潔さに驚く人が少なくありません。感染症予防の立場からも、清潔という概念は、鍼灸の臨床では基本的で非常に重要な要素となります。

そして、日本の保健所の指導や日本人の専門家の臨床現場では、清潔で衛生的ということが徹底されています。その典型的な例として、日本の臨床現場では、ステンレス製ディスポーザブル鍼灸針が針の主流となっています。

鍼の施術では、針を体内に刺入する行為が行われることから、鍼灸の臨床現場では、HIV、B型肝炎・C型肝炎などに対する感染予防対策が重要な課題となります。

日本では、従来は高圧滅菌器で滅菌作業を行うことで、針は何度も繰り返して使用されていました。しかし、感染に対する懸念から、高圧滅菌器で完全滅菌したとしても、針を使い回すことに対して、不安感や抵抗感を感じる利用者も少なくありません。このような事情から、日本では世界に先駆けて、単回使用を目的としたステンレス製の「ディスポーザブル鍼灸針」が開発されました。

ディスポーザブル鍼灸針は、日本の鍼灸針のトップメーカーである「セイリン株式会社」（以下：セイリン）が開発し、1978年より販売が開始されました。セイリンによれば、現在、日本国内では、推定で全体の80％以上の臨床現場で、ステンレス製ディスポーザブル鍼灸針が使用されているということです。

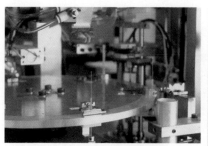

ディスポーザブル鍼灸針の製造過程
（セイリン提供）

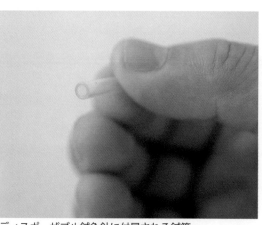

ディスポーザブル鍼灸針に付属される鍼管

完全滅菌の状態で出荷され、使い捨てで使用するディスポーザブル鍼灸針は、日本国内ばかりでなく、世界各地から強く求められるようになり、セイリンは、ヨーロッパとアメリカを中心に、積極的に針の輸出を行ってきました。

日本発のディスポーザブル鍼灸針は世界各地において針のイメージを変え、鍼の需要を大幅に拡大させました。反対に、今の時代にディスポーザブル鍼灸針が存在していなければ、鍼治療は大幅に衰退していた可能性も考えられます。

日本の「単回使用」の針という発想と製造技術は、鍼の臨床における衛生面の不安と問題を大幅に改善し、鍼治療の普及と需要の拡大に多大な貢献を果たしました。ステンレス製のディスポーザブル鍼灸針は、現在では世界中の多くの国々で広く普及し、鍼灸針の主流となりました。

鍼の技術面からばかりでなく、針の品質と性能の向上という面から、鍼の健全な普及と発展に取り組んできたことも、日本鍼灸の大きな特徴です。

そして、セイリンが日本の針のメーカーであることから、セイリンが製造する針は、針体が細くてプラスチック製の単回使用の鍼管が付属しているの日本仕様です。したがって、現在、世界各地に細いディスポーザブル鍼灸針と管鍼法が普及したことには、セイリンの針の輸出に対する企業努

力も少なからず関与していると考えられます。

このように、ディスポーザブル鍼灸針は、日本の針メーカーの発明品であり、Shinkyu の清潔で衛生的という特徴を象徴するものです。そればかりでなく、日本の Shinkyu の臨床現場では、様々な器具、タオル、施術着などの全てにおいて、清潔で衛生的ということに対して細かく配慮されており、利用者の方々から高く評価されています。

◆ 洗練性

日本の伝統的な文化、宗教、知識、技術などの多くは、日本人がゼロから生み出したものではなく、中国から伝来し、長い時間の中で、日本人の特性を通じて変化を遂げたものです。

このような事実は、日本人が「質」や「完成度」を高めることに優れ、物事を洗練することが得意なことを示唆しています。日本人には、0から1を生む能力には乏しく不得手な傾向がありますが、一方で、1を100どころか1000にまで高める能力を有しているということでしょう。

鍼灸も、日本人がゼロから生み出したものではなく、古代の中国に発祥した針灸が6世紀に伝来したものです。そして、日本人は長い時間をかけて様々な独創的な手法や道具を生み出し、また、針灸を洗練して、上記のような独自性と洗練性を有する「日本鍼灸」を作り上げたのです。

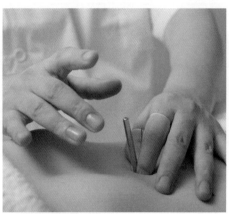

日本鍼灸を象徴する管鍼法

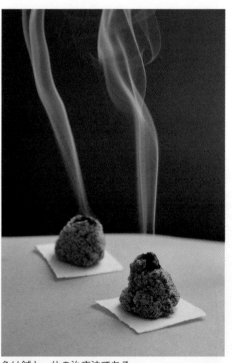

灸は鍼と一体の治療法である

世界的規模で見た場合には、現状では、臨床現場で実践されている鍼灸の主流は中国式の針灸であり、日本鍼灸を実践する専門家は少数派です。つまり、「量」の面では、今のところは日本鍼灸に優位性はありません。

しかし一方で、上記のように、丁寧、繊細、衛生的などの理由から、日本の鍼灸は、「質」の面で優れた特徴、優位性、信頼性を持つ洗練された鍼灸として世界各地で評価されており、学校教育は中国式であっても、臨床現場では、日本式の丁寧で繊細な鍼灸を実践したいという専門家がますます増えています。

そして、このような日本鍼灸を象徴する技術と道具として位置付けられているのが、管鍼法、細い針、ディスポーザブル鍼灸針です。そこで、日本において鍼術が開花した17世紀にさかのぼり、鍼術の健全な普及と発展に生涯を捧げた杉山和一の実像に迫り、彼の思想、知識、技術、功績について学んでいきましょう。

Chapter

3

鍼術と気

◆気を診て、気を操る

杉山和一は、鍼術において、「気」という存在を特に重視していました。東洋の伝統医学の根底には、気という存在があり、気は、鍼術の治療の基本とされてきたからです。

『杉山真伝流』の表之巻第四および皆伝之巻では、「気を診て、気を操ることが鍼術の目的である」と説かれており、鍼術を行う者が気を感得することの重要性が繰り返し強調されています。

気には、正反対の性質を持つ2種類のものがあるとされています。

一つは、生命体が生命活動を正常に維持していくために必要な生体エネルギーであり、「真気」と呼ばれています。真気は、人体を構成する最も基本的で重要な物質とされ、「正気」とも呼ばれます。

もう一つは、正常な生命活動を阻害する負のエネルギーであり、「邪気」と呼ばれています。邪気には、体外から侵入する「風邪」「寒邪」「暑邪」「湿邪」「燥邪」「熱邪」の6種類の「外邪」と、情動の乱れから体内で発生するものがあるとされています。

「気」という言葉が単独で用いられる場合には、通常は、このうちの真気を指します。気は、体内において、「経絡」という通り道を通じて全身をくまなく循環しているとされています。経絡は、東洋の伝統医学特有の概念であり、西洋の現代医学に同様の概念は存在しません。そして、気も経絡も目視できるものではありません。

「経絡」の「経」とは、縦に通る主要な太い通り道、「絡」とは、横に通る細い通り道を意味しています。経絡を、道路にたとえれば、「幹線道路」と一般の「道路」や「道」の全てによる交通ネットワークであり、このネットワー

30

クを利用すれば、日本全国どこへでも行くことができます。気は、このような経絡を通じて全身をくまなく循環しており、体中のどこにでも存在しています。

そして、気は、同じく人体を構成する基本物質である「血（けつ）」を引っぱりながら、人体を循環しているとされています。

伝統医学では、邪気を除去し、真気の正常な活動を維持、増進することが、健康の維持、増進、回復をはか

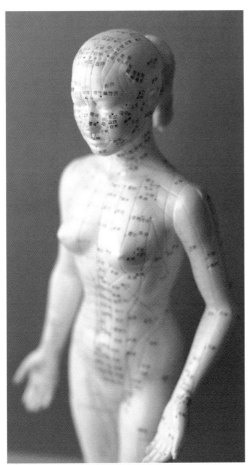

気は経絡を通って全身にくまなく巡っている

ることであると考えられています。

例えば、外敵の攻撃を受けたり、内紛が起きたりして、町が戦争状態になってしまった場合には、最初に敵を撃退し、その後に物資と食糧を供給して復旧作業を行うことで、平和な日常生活を取り戻すことができます。人間の体においては、この場合の敵に相当するものが「邪気」であり、物資と食糧に相当するものが「真気」と「血」という存在です。

現代では、日本においても、西洋の現代医学が医学の主流となり、医療現場では、気の存在が忘れ去られている傾向があります。同様に、鍼灸の教育現場や臨床現場においても、解剖学や生理学などの現代医学的な知識が重視されるようになり、気に対する認識はますます希薄になっています。

しかし、鍼術は本来、伝統医学の主要な治療法であり、鍼灸が発祥した古代の中国においても、杉山和一が活躍した17世紀の日本においても、西洋医学的な知識や認識は存在せず、鍼術は伝統医学の理論を基盤として実践されていました。そして、目には見えない気を診て、気を操ることが、鍼術の真髄であると認識されていました。

一方、現代では、このような認識はおおよそ重視されなくなりましたが、時代が変わっても、伝統医学を基盤として発展してきた鍼の施術では、西洋の現代医学的な知識や認識が全てではありません。杉山和一の鍼術を学ぶことで、「気を診て、気を操ることが鍼術の目的である」という鍼術の基本思想を再認識することができます。そして、鍼術を行う者にとって、気の存在を認識することが、いかに重要なことであるかを理解することができるでしょう。

◆ 気に対する鍼術の作用

『杉山真伝流』を紐解くことで、鍼術は、気に対して、「響き」「補法」「瀉法」「誘導」「調和」の五つの重要な作用があることを理解できます。

その中でも特に、刺針によって引き起こされる「響き」という現象によって「気を至らせる」ということが、鍼術の治療効果にとって基本的で不可欠な要素であることが説明されています。

◎ 作用① 「響き」～気を至らせる～

体に針を刺すことによって、患者が感じる独特の感覚を、中国では「得気」、日本では「響き」と呼んでいます。

「得気」と「響き」は、同義語として認識される場合もありますが、類似した感覚でありながら、全く同じではないという認識もあります。

得気と響きは、いずれも体に針を刺すことによって生じる患者の「生体反応」であることに相違はありませんが、一般に、響きは得気よりも穏やかで軽い反応であると認識されています。その要因は、使用される針の太さと刺針法の違いによるものであろうと考えられます。

中国では日本で一般的に使用されている針よりも太い針を、「捻針法」と呼ばれる刺針法を用いて一気に刺針します。捻針法は、母指と示指で針柄を持ち、針を素速く回転させながら、皮膚に対して直接刺針する技法です。得気とは、この場合に、患者が刺針部位に感じる「酸」（だるいような感覚）、「脹」（腫れぼったいような感覚）、「重」（重だるいような感覚）、「麻」（しびれたような感覚）の感覚であると定義されています。

一方、日本では、中国で一般的に使用されている針よりも細い針を、管鍼法を用いて穏やかに刺針するため、

それぞれの刺針を受けた場合の患者の生体反応は異なる可能性があります。したがって、響きという感覚は、管鍼法と細い針が創案されたことで、日本で生まれた日本鍼灸特有の感覚といえます。管鍼法と細い針によって生じる患者の生体反応は、「響き」として認識することが必要です。

気に対する認識が希薄となった現在では、鍼灸の教育現場や臨床現場において、得気や響きという現象に対する認識と理解も希薄になっています。得気は「気至」とも呼ばれ、「気を至らせる」ことを目的として、刺針によって引き起こされる生体反応であるとされています。

中国では古来より、得気は鍼術の治療効果を左右する重要な現象であると認識されてきました。中国から伝来した鍼術を学んだ杉山和一も、気を至らせることを重視しており、「針を刺す時は、気を察し、気を至らせることが重要で、治療効果を得ることができるかどうかは唯一これによる」と説いています。このことは、「治療効果を得るためには気を至らせることが重要である」ということであると同時に、「気を至らせることができなければ治療効果を得ることはできない」ということを示唆しています。

得気と響きは、「刺針によって治療効果を得るための最初の生体反応」であり、同時に「気を至らせることを目的として引き起こされる刺針による生体反応」として理解することができます。

「至らせる」とは、その場所に「行き届かせる」「行き渡らせる」という意味の言葉です。そして、「気を至らせる」ということには、狭義と広義の二つの意味があります。

狭義には、「患部局所に真気を至らせる」ことであり、「刺針した針の針尖に響きを感じること」です。例えば、邪気に阻害されて真気が巡っていないことが原因で疼痛がある場合に、刺針によって邪気を除去し、真気

34

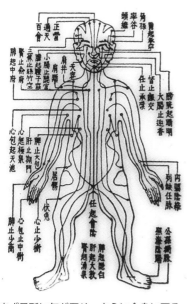

まず局所に気が至り、さらに全身に至る

を至らせることで、疼痛を緩和できるということです。

広義には、「全身に真気が巡って爽快感を感じること」です。

『霊枢』九鍼十二原篇には、「気を至らせる」ということについて、「刺針の要点は、気が至ってこそ効果がある。効果が得られた場合の感覚は、風が雲を吹き散らして、蒼天を見るようなものである」という内容の記載が見られます。

一方、「邪気は針先に至り来るのが速く、至ると針下にピリピリとした緊張を感じる。これに反して、真気は針先に至り来るのが遅く、ゆっくり至るとともに針下が温まり柔和に感じる」という記載もあり、真気が刺針した針の針尖に至るのには一定の時間がかかることが説明されています。

そして、真気が局所ばかりでなく全身に巡るのにはさらに時間がかかることから、鍼の響きとは、局所に気を至らせることであると同時に、それを起点として、患部局所と全身に対してさらに気を巡らせ、至らせるための最初の生体反応であると理解されます。つまり、響きという生体反応が生じることで、気は、時間の経過とともに、局所、そしてさらには全身に至るということです。

反対に、響きを得ることができなかった場合には、

35

気は、局所にも全身にも至ることができることはなく、治療効果も得ることができないということです。

また、気を至らせることができたかどうかは、患部においては、「針下が温まり柔和に感じる」ことが指標となり、全身においては、「爽快感を感じること」が指標になると理解することができます。私たちは、刺針後に「置針」を行う場合がありますが、最近まで置針の意味について深く考えたことがありませんでした。しかし、「真気が至るのは遅い」ということを学ぶことで、置針の目的を理解することができました。

◎作用② 「補法」 〜気血を巡らせる〜

何らかの原因によって、道路や道の人通りが長期的に少なくなると、その周辺の町は、全体的にさびれていく結果となります。同様に、人体では経絡を循環する気が不足した場合にも、体調に何らかの悪影響を及ぼします。

そして、気が局所的に不足している場合には、その局所に針を刺すことで、気を巡らせ、不足した気を補うことが鍼術の目的となります。

また、伝統医学の理論では、気が血を引っぱって体内を循環していると認識されていることから、気が巡れば血も巡ると考えられています。

◎作用③ 「瀉法」 〜邪気を発散させる〜

道路の交通が渋滞した場合と同様に、経絡を循環する気が渋滞すると、滞った気は、「気滞（きたい）」という邪気に相当する病理産物となり、やはり体調に何らかの悪影響を及ぼします。

そして、気が局所的に滞っている場合には、その局所に針を刺すことで、滞った気を散らすことが鍼術の目

的となります。

同様に、外邪が体内に侵入して真気の活動を阻害している場合にも、針を刺すことで邪気を除去し、気血を巡らせることが鍼術の目的となります。

◎ 作用④ 「誘導」 ～気を経絡の末端、表裏関係の部位に誘導する～

例えば、体幹部に邪気が存在して疼痛を引き起こしている場合には、患部の局所と関連する経絡の手足末端の経穴に針を刺すことで、邪気を末端におびき寄せ、患部の疼痛を軽減させることができます。

また例えば、腹部の病変に対して、背部に針を刺すことで、「裏」から「表」に気を誘導し、症状を改善することができます。

このように、邪気を誘導させることを目的とした別の部位に対する意図的な刺針は、「引き鍼」と呼ばれています。

◎ 作用⑤ 「調和」 ～気血を調和させる～

「調和」とは、「全体がほどよくつりあって、矛盾や衝突などがなく、和合している状態」という意味であり、究極的に平和な状態を意味しています。これを人体に当てはめると、「全身がほどよくつりあっている状態」であると理解できます。

一方、東洋の伝統医学は陰陽の調和を重視しており、健康状態とは、陰陽の調和が保たれている状態であると認識されています。気血は、人体を構成し生命活動を維持するための基本物質であり、気は「陽気」とも呼

ばれて「陽」、血は「陰血」とも呼ばれて「陰」であるとされています。したがって、気血の調和を保つことが、健康状態を維持するための基本となります。

一方、鍼術の「響き」「補法」「瀉法」「誘導」の目的を掘り下げて考えると、気血の「調和」をはかることが目的であると考えられます。局所と全身の気血を調和させるために、必要に応じて、気を至らせ、邪気を除去し、気血を巡らせるということです。

鍼の施術後に患者が「体が軽くなった」「気持ちが良くて寝てしまった」など、術後の爽快感を表現する場合がありますが、これは、全身の気血が調和した結果、全身の気血が調和した状態を示唆しています。

針の要点は、気が至ってこそ効果がある。効果が得られた場合の感覚は、風が雲を吹き散らして、蒼天を見るようなものである」という記載も、全身の気血が調和した状態を示唆しています。

このように、鍼術の本来の目的は、真気の過不足や邪気の存在を特定し、「響き」「補法」「瀉法」「誘導」の四つの作用を臨機応変に操ることで、気を至らせ、邪気を除去し、気血を巡らせ、気血を「調和」させることです。

そして、真気も邪気も目で見ることができないため、鍼術を行う者は、気を「感得する」ことが必要となります。『杉山真伝流』の表之巻第四、および皆伝之巻において強調されているように、杉山和一の鍼術を学ぶ上では「気を診て、気を操ること」という鍼術の基本思想を再認識することが必要となります。

Chapter 4

刺針法としての管鍼法

◆世界標準の刺針法へ

本書の冒頭で述べたとおり管鍼法は、広義には、単なる刺針法ではなく、管鍼術を含めた「鍼管を用いた鍼術の技法全般」であり、狭義には、「鍼管を用いた刺針法」です。

本章では、管鍼法を刺針法と管鍼術に分類し、それぞれの技法について解説していきます。

管鍼法は、鍼管と呼ばれる補助器具を用いる刺針の技法であり、「管鍼法」という用語は、一般的には、この刺針法としての狭義の管鍼法を指します。

管鍼法では、極めて細い針でも容易に刺針を行うことができることから、日本では、教育現場においても臨床現場においても、標準的な刺針法となっています。そして、現在では、日本国内ばかりでなく、海外の諸外国においても、多くの専門家がこの技法によって刺針を行っており、世界的にも標準的な刺針法になりつつあります。

◆鍼管

日本では現在、ステンレス製のディスポーザブル鍼灸針が主流となっています。ディスポーザブル鍼灸針には、プラスティック製のディスポーザブル鍼管が同梱されています。そのため、針も鍼管も単回使用となります。しかし従来は、ステンレスや銀の鍼管が標準的に使用されていました。

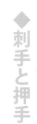

◆刺手と押手

中国由来の撚針法では、刺針は片手で行われます。一方、管鍼法では、利き手と反対の手で、鍼管と刺針部位の針を保持した状態で刺針が行われます。この場合に、針を刺入する利き手は「刺手」、鍼管と刺針部位の針を保持する手は「押手」と呼ばれます。

杉山真伝流には、十四種類の押手があり、状況に応じて使い分けられていました。しかし、着衣の上から刺

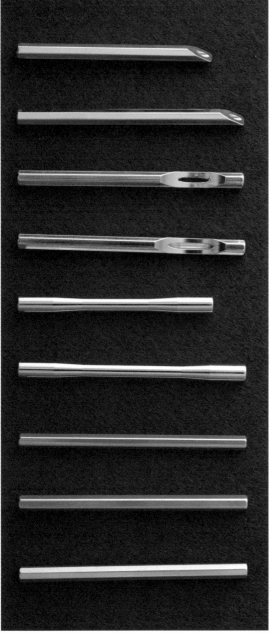

様々な鍼管〈実物大〉

満月の押手

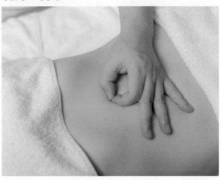

小指側の手掌を皮膚にピタッと付け、母指と示指で円をつくり、指端はきつくつまむ。残りの3指はまっすぐに伸ばし皮膚に付ける。針を直刺する時に用いる押手。

半月の押手

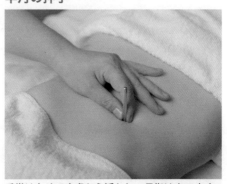

手掌は丸めて皮膚から浮かし、母指はまっすぐに伸ばして皮膚に付け、示指は丸めて半円をつくる。残りの3指は伸ばすが、狭い部位ではたたむこともある。針を斜刺する時に用いる押手。

針する場合の押手など、現代では実用的でないものもあります。

現在は、「満月の押手」「半月の押手」と呼ばれる押手が、一般的に用いられています。

◆挿管

刺針を行うために、針を鍼管に挿入する過程を「挿管（そうかん）」といいます。挿管には、両手で行う「両手挿管法」と片手で行う「片手挿管法」の2種類の方法があります。

現在、日本の針の主流となっているディスポーザブル鍼灸針は、予め付属のディスポーザブル鍼管に挿入されているものが多いことから、挿管の過程は不要になりつつあります。

両手挿管法

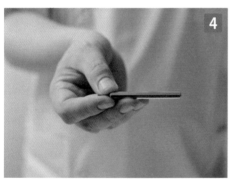

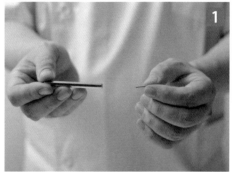

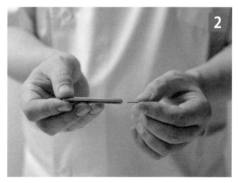

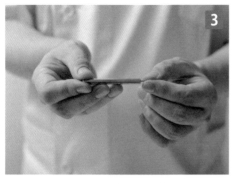

①押手に鍼管を持ち、刺手に針柄をつまみ持つ。
②針柄を管先に近づける。
③針柄から針を管の中に入れる。
④少し管を立てれば針全体が管に収まる。管頭から出てきた針柄を母指と示指でつまむ。

◎両手挿管法

　押手に鍼管を持ち、刺手に針柄を持ちます。針を針柄から鍼管に挿入し、鍼管の管頭側から突出した針柄を、刺手の母指と示指で固定します。

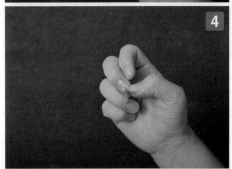

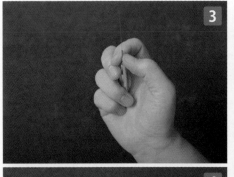

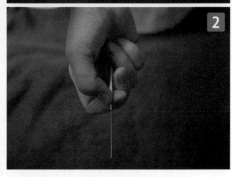

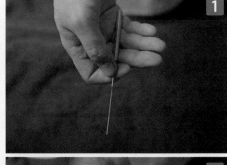

①鍼管を手掌に収め、母指と示指で針柄をつまむ。
②針柄から針を管先に入れる。
③管を立て、鍼を鍼管の中に収める。
④中指を鍼管の中央部に当てる。
⑤中指を支点として管を半回転させる。
⑥母指と示指とで管頭と針柄とをつまむ。

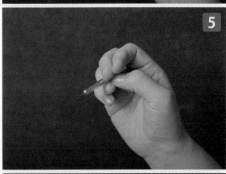

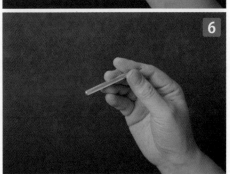

◎片手挿管法

刺手だけで行う挿管の技法であり、日本で最も一般的に行われている挿管法です。初心者にとっては比較的に難易度が高い技法であり、練習が必要とされます。

日本の鍼灸師の養成施設では、片手挿管法を習得することが必須とされています。

◆切皮・弾入

◎切皮

「切皮(せっぴ)」とは、針が皮膚に侵入するために針尖が表皮を破る過程です。「弾入(だんにゅう)」とは、管鍼法における切皮の技法です。

◎弾入

刺針部位の皮膚の上で、針が挿管された鍼管を押手の母指と示指で支持します。刺手を鍼管から離して、刺手の示指で鍼管から突出した針柄の後部を軽く叩きます。

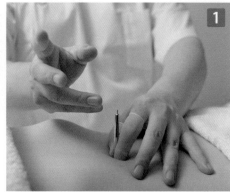

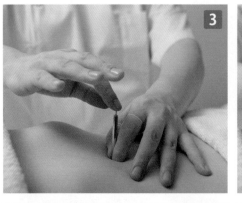

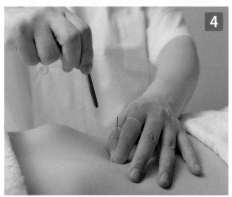

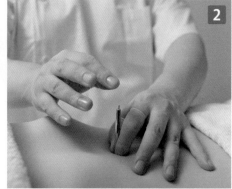

①押手の母指と示指で針の挿入された鍼管を皮膚上に立てる。

②針柄は管頭から3mmほど出ている。

③針柄の頭を軽く3〜5回に分けて叩く。

④押手の母指と示指で刺入された針をつまんだまま、鍼管を抜き去る。

◎刺入

日本において、針を刺入する一般的な方法は2種類あります。

● 送り込み刺法

刺手の母指と示指で針柄を持ち、適切な圧力を加えて針を皮下に送り込むように刺入します。

送り込み刺法

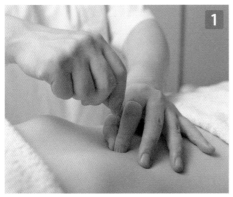

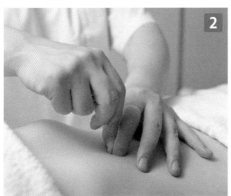

①押手の母指と示指で針体をつまみ、刺手で針柄をつまむ。
②刺手の母指と示指を段階的に伸ばしつつ、針を刺入する。

旋撚刺法

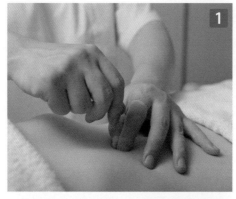

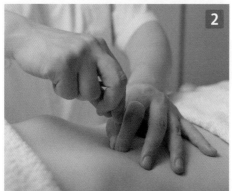

①針柄をつまんだ刺手の母指と示指をすべらせ、
　針を右回転させる。
②同じく針を左回転させる。右と左と回転をくり
　返しながら、針を刺入する。

● 旋撚刺法

刺手の母指と示指で針柄を持ち、針尖を右または左に120度から180度程度回転させながら刺入します。

Chapter 5

十四管術の実践

◆十四管術の目的と分類

杉山和一が考案した十四管術は、いずれも、刺針部位に対して付加的な刺激を与えるために鍼管を用いる技法であり、十四種類の術式があることから、十四管術と呼ばれています。

十四管術の主な目的と作用は、刺針による「響き」「補法」「瀉法」「誘導」「調和」の作用を「増強」し、また、刺針部位の周囲に、響きと刺激を「伝播」することで、刺針による治療効果を高めることです。

① 増強：刺針の効果を増強する
② 伝播：刺針部の周囲に響きと刺激を伝える

◎十四管術の目的

十四管術は、その術式によって大きく4種類に分類することができます。本章では、十四管術を4種類に分類し、その特徴と臨床応用について解説し、それぞれの術の主な作用、技法、『杉山真伝流』に記載されている具体的な使用例についても記載します。

また、十四管術を技法と目的に基づいて分析すると、技法に若干の相違はあるものの、同類と認められる術が存在します。そして、同類の術の共通性と相違点を認識することで、それぞれの術の作用と使用目的を、より明確に理解することができ、臨床応用に役立てることができます。

そこで本章では、十四管術のそれぞれの術の共通性についても解説します。

◎十四管術の分類

十四管術の四つの分類は以下となります。　以降、それぞれの詳細について詳しくご説明していきます。

① 針とともに叩く術

細指管、暁の管、気拍管

② 針とともに推す術

推指管、爻延管

③ 針の周囲を叩く、摩擦する術

扣管、撥指管、遠覚管、随肉管

④ 針を振動させる術

竜頭管、巧指管、犢鍼管、内調管、通谷管

◆ ① 針とともに叩く術

細指管、暁の管、気拍管

【主な作用】

針とともに叩く術は、技法は類似していますが、それぞれの術の主な目的は異なります。

細指管：表層の邪熱を発散します（瀉法）。

暁の管：深部に鬱滞している邪熱を引き出して発散します（瀉法）。

気拍管：刺針部位の周囲に響きを伝播します（調和）。

【共通性と相違点】

細指管も暁の管も、管を針にはめた状態で上部を叩く技法は共通していますが、細指管は管頭から突出している針柄（竜頭）の頭を叩くのに対し、暁の管は2段階に刺入した針に管をはめて管頭を叩くところが異なります。

また、気拍管では、刺入した針に管を添えて、その管頭を叩きます。

◎ 細指管（さいしかん）　Fine Finger Kan

● 名称の由来

鍼管から突出している針柄の頭を細かくリズミカルに叩くことから、この技法は細指管と名付けられた。

● 主な作用

皮下の表層に鬱滞する邪気を発散させる（瀉法）。

● 鍼管の持ち方

針を挿入した状態で、押手の母指と示指で鍼管の管先を持つ。

● 技法

針と鍼管を施術部位に当て、鍼管から突出した針柄（竜頭）の頭を示指で100〜200回ほど細かく叩く。

叩く回数が多いほど良い。

終了後は、針、鍼管、押手ともに皮膚から離し、別の施術部位に当て、同様に示指で針柄の頭を細かく叩く。

● 使用例

感冒によって悪寒がして発熱し、頚・肩・背・腰がこわばって痛む場合に、患部に用いる（瀉法）。

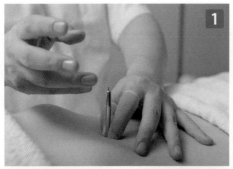

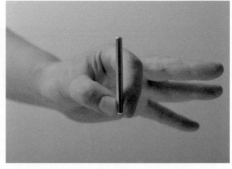

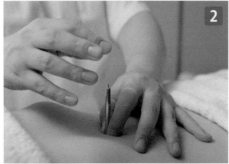

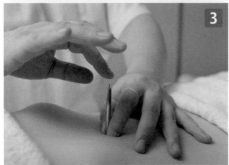

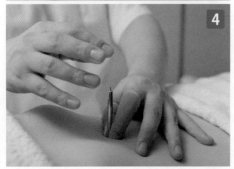

【持ち方】 管先を押手の母指と示指でつまむ。

①針の挿入された鍼管を押手でつまみ、皮膚に当てる。
②管頭から3mmほど出ている針柄の頭。
③刺手の示指頭で針柄の頭を軽く叩く。
④示指頭を針柄の頭から離し、また軽く叩く。これを100回ほど細かく続ける。

皮膚や表層筋の緊張をゆるめ、発汗を促し、風寒湿の外邪を発散させたい場合に、僧帽筋全体に用いる（瀉法）。

目に涙が出て痛痒く目の中に赤い細脈がある場合に、攢竹に用いる（瀉法）。

血が鬱滞して月経不調となった場合に、照海や至陰に用いる（誘導）。

産後に胸腹が痛む場合に、内関に用いる（誘導）。

◎　暁の管　Rising sun Kan
あかつき　くだ

● 名称の由来

朝日が昇るように、鍼管を叩いて深部の邪熱を段階的に引き上げることから、この術は暁の管と名付けられた。

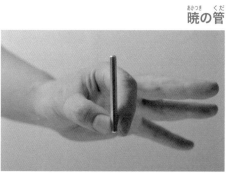

暁の管
あかつき　くだ

【持ち方】　管先を押手の母指と示指でつまむ。

● 主な作用

深層に鬱滞した邪気を表層へと引き出し、発散させる（瀉法）。

響きを促し、気血を巡らせる（補法）。

虚実にかかわらず、疼痛全般に用いる。

● 鍼管の持ち方

管を針にはめた状態で、押手の母指と示指で鍼管の管先を持つ。

● 技法

針と鍼管を刺針部位に当て弾入し、鍼管を取り除いて針を二、三分（約5ミリ）刺入したら、再び鍼管を針にはめ、細指管のように細かく管頭を叩く。

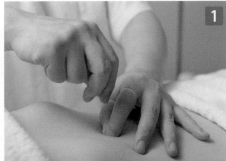

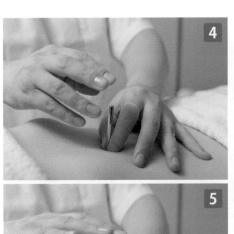

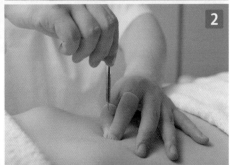

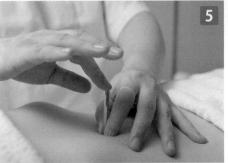

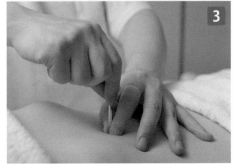

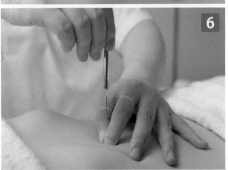

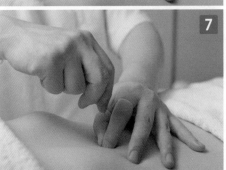

①針を約5mm刺入する。
②刺入した針に針柄から鍼管をはめる。
③はめた管を皮膚に当てる。
④刺手の示指頭で、
⑤管頭を叩く。この動作を30〜50回くり返す。
⑥鍼管を抜き去る。
⑦針をさらに約5mm刺入する。

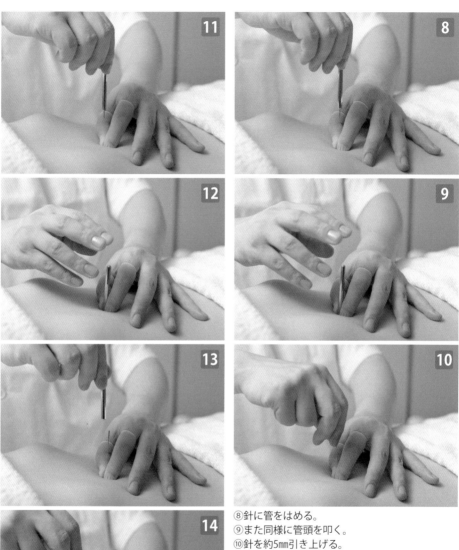

⑧針に管をはめる。
⑨また同様に管頭を叩く。
⑩針を約5mm引き上げる。
⑪針に管をはめる。
⑫また同様に管頭を叩く。
⑬鍼管を抜き去る。
⑭針も抜き去る。

再び鍼管を取り除いて針を二、三分（約5ミリ）刺入して鍼管を針にはめ、同様に細かく管頭を叩く。

このようにして、同じ動作を2、3回繰り返し、目標とする深度まで刺入する。

抜針時も、二、三分引いては、管頭を細かく叩き、最後に一分（約2ミリ）ほど抜いて細かく叩いた後に抜針する。

暁の管は、今日でいう「示指打法」を段階的に用いる技法である。

● 使用例

四肢の疼痛、関節の炎症による疼痛に対して、熱邪を発散させる（瀉法）。

月経不調や生理痛、食欲不振の場合に、腹部あるいは背腰部に用いる（瀉法＋補法）。

胸腹部に疼痛や邪気がある場合に、関連する経絡の末端の穴に邪気を誘導する（誘導）。

足の麻痺に対して、陰陵泉に用いる（補法）。

足の内側や足底が痛む場合に、公孫と湧泉を治療した上で、足の血流を促す目的で足三里に用いる（補法）。

傷寒の陰証の場合に、関元に用いる（補法）。

しゃっくりが止まらない場合に、上脘に用いる（補法）。

虚寒で下痢する場合に、天枢に用いる（補法）。

産後に血塊があり腹痛がする場合に、腹部の気を調えた上で、三陰交に用いて腹部の邪気を下へと引き下ろす（誘導）。

◎気拍管（きはくかん）　Ki-tapping Kan

●名称の由来

気を至らせることを目的として、鍼管で皮膚を細かく叩く（＝拍）ことから、この技法は気拍管と名付けられた。

●主な作用

響きを促した後に、深部に鬱滞した気を浮かせ、周囲に響きを伝える（調和）。

大きな筋肉の筋緊張をゆるめる（補法）。

●鍼管の持ち方

最初に押手の母指と示指で、鍼管の管先を持つ。

●技法

針を目標とする深度まで直刺で刺入し、満月の押手の母指と示指を少し開いて鍼管を針の傍に当て、管頭を細指術のように細かく叩く（響き）。

3〜4呼吸ほど止めたら鍼管を取り除き、少し針を浮かせ、また別の方向から鍼管を針の傍に当て、鍼管を細かく叩く。上下左右の四方から、同様にこれを行う。

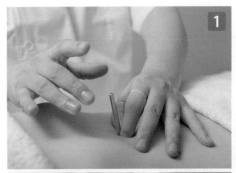

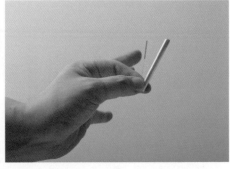

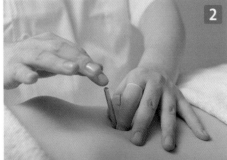

【持ち方】 針に管を添えて、針先と管先の両方を
母指と示指でつまむ。

①刺入した針に鍼管を添えて、母指と示指の間に
鍼管を挟み立てる。
②管頭を刺手の示指頭で細かく叩く。
③次に示指と中指の間に鍼管を挟み立てる。
④同様に管頭を細かく叩く。

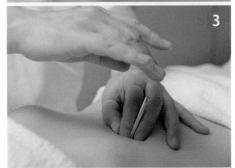

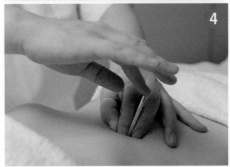

これは気を周囲にまで至らせることが目的である。叩き終わって鍼管を取り除いたら、直ちに抜針する。

● **使用例**

上腹部の痛み、側頭部の痛み、四肢の厥冷や転筋など、炎症や冷えによる筋緊張、疼痛に用い、また、背部
兪穴、側頭筋（角孫）、足底筋（湧泉）、大腿筋膜張筋（風市）など幅の広い筋肉に用いる。

産後に出血が止まらない場合に、肝の機能を調える目的で、膈兪と肝兪に用いる（調和）。

膝が曲がって筋肉が引きつり痛む場合に、風市に用いる（補法）。

足が痛む場合に、湧泉に用いる（瀉法）。

虫歯が痛む場合に、角孫に用いる（瀉法）。

虚した臓腑の機能を調えるために、背部兪穴に用いる（補法）。

 ②針とともに推す術

【主な作用】

推指管、爻延管

針尖が届かない深部の筋緊張や硬結をゆるめ、気血を巡らせます（瀉法＋補法）。

【臨床応用】

患者が敏感なために深く刺入できない場合や、初めて鍼治療を受ける若い患者に用います。針を浅めに刺入した上で、針尖部よりも深い部位にある筋緊張や硬結をゆるめたい場合に用いると効果的です。

【共通性と相違点】

鍼管を針にはめて鍼管を針とともに推すか（推指管）、鍼管を針に添わせて鍼管を針とともに推すか（爻綖管）、

推指管と爻綖管は同類の術であり、両者の違いは、鍼管を針に添わせて鍼管を針とともに推すか（爻綖管）の違いで、目的と作用は同じです。

◎ 推指管　<ruby>推<rt>すい</rt></ruby><ruby>指<rt>し</rt></ruby><ruby>管<rt>かん</rt></ruby>　Finger pressing Kan

● 名称の由来

指で針と鍼管を細かく推すことから、この術は推指管と名付けられた。

● 主な作用

邪気を発散させる（瀉法）。

気血を巡らせる（補法）。

推指管
すいしかん

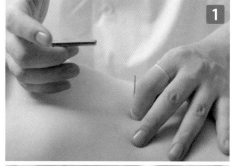

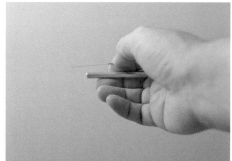

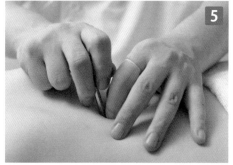

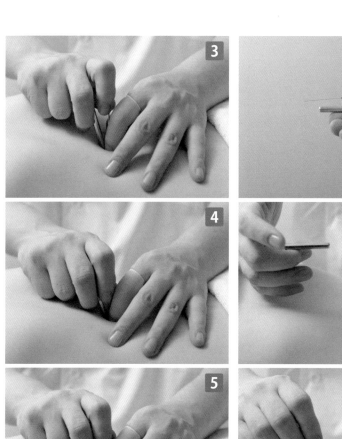

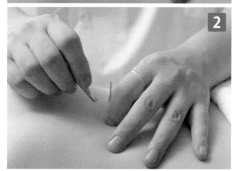

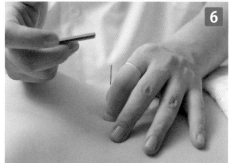

【持ち方】　母指と示指で針柄を持ち、中指の付け
　根の関節横紋に管頭を挟む。

①目的の深さまで針を刺入する。
②針に添えて管先を皮膚に当てる。
③刺手の母指と示指で針柄を持ち、中指で管を持
　つ。
④針と管とを同時に推し、
⑤また戻す。この推したり戻したりする動作をく
　り返す。
⑥目的を果たしたら、管を取り除き、針も抜く。

● 鍼管の持ち方

押手の母指と示指で鍼管の管先を持ち、刺手の母指と示指で針柄を持ち、中指の付け根の関節横紋に管頭をはさむ。

● 技法

針を目標とする深度よりやや浅く直刺し、針に沿わせて鍼管を皮膚に当て、管先を押手ではさむ。

刺手の母指と示指で針柄（竜頭）を持ち、中指の付け根の関節横紋に鍼頭をはさみ、押手と刺手をそろえて鍼管を針とともに数十回推す。

● 使用例

腹部が冷えて悪風がする時に、中脘に用いる（補法）。

膀胱炎にて下腹部が熱痛し、小便が赤くなり、気滞して下腹部や腰がかき乱されるように痛む場合に、下腹部や腰の穴に用いる（瀉法）。

臍下痛に対して、三陰交と陰陵泉に用いる（誘導）。

両肘とも引きつる場合に、上廉に用いる（補法）。

◎交泛管　Tube pressing Kan
(こうしょかん)

●名称の由来

「爻」とは、易の陰と陽の卦を組み立てることで、「交わる」という意味である。「泛」とは、「通る」「達する」という意味である。

針（＝陽）に管（＝陰）を交え、気を通すことを目的として、上下に揺さぶることから、この術は交泛管と名付けられた。

●主な作用

筋緊張、硬結をゆるめる（瀉法＋補法）。

●鍼管の持ち方

押手の母指と示指で鍼管の管先を持ち、刺手の母指と示指で鍼管の上部をつまみ、中指と薬指を管に添える。

●技法

目的とする深度まで刺針したら、針に鍼管をはめて管先を皮膚に当て、これを数十回推す。そして、鍼管を取り除き、針で雀啄や旋捻などの手技を行ったら、再び鍼管をはめて、これを数十回推す。

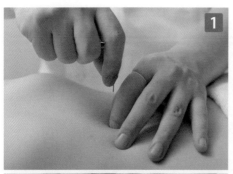

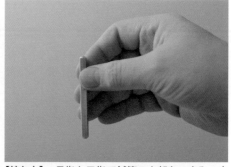

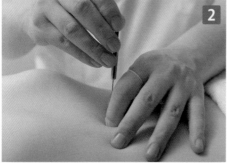

こうしょかん
交竧管

【持ち方】　母指と示指で鍼管の上部をつまみ、中指と薬指を管に添え、小指は薬指に添える。

①針を刺入する。
②刺入した針の針柄頭から管をはめる。
③鍼管を皮膚に当てる。
④押手とともに管先で皮膚を推しては戻す。この動作をくり返す。

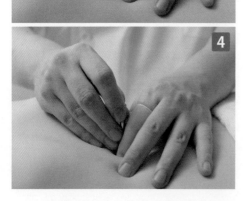

● 使用例

　若い患者で、眼精疲労のため頚肩がこわばっている場合に、筋緊張や硬結をゆるめる目的で用いる（補法）。

　敏感な患者で、腹痛・背痛・腰痛などによる深部の筋緊張や硬結をゆるめる目的で用いる（補法＋瀉法）。

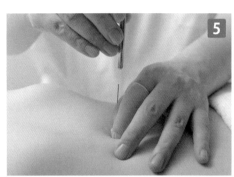

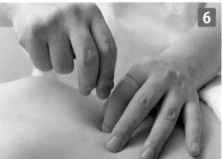

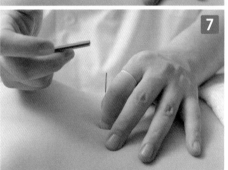

⑤目的を果たしたら、管を取り去る。
⑥刺入してある針を持ち、雀啄や旋撚などの手技
　を行う。その後、再び管をはめ、管で推し戻す
　動作をくり返す（②～④）。
⑦目的を果たしたら、管を取り除き、針も抜く。

◆ ③針の周囲を叩く、摩擦する術

扣管、撥指管、遠覚管、随肉管

【主な作用】
①邪気を発散させ、筋緊張をゆるめ、疼痛を軽減させます（瀉法）。
②刺針部の周囲に気血を集めて筋緊張をゆるめます（補法）。

【臨床応用】

気滞や邪熱が皮膚や筋肉の表層に広く存在して痛む場合に用います。

扣管・撥指管・遠覚管は、主に、邪気が実している疼痛部位に用います。また、気が虚して冷えている部位にも用います。その場合には、ゆっくりと推すように叩くことで、冷えた筋緊張をゆるめ、気血を巡らすことができます。

遠覚管は瀉法の効果を増強する目的で用い、随肉管は補法の効果を増強する目的で用いるところが異なります。

【術の分類】

①針の周囲を叩く術……扣管、撥指管、遠覚管
②針の周囲を摩擦する術……随肉管

【共通性と相違点】

●扣管・撥指管

扣管と撥指管は同類の術であり、両者の違いは、刺入した針の周囲の皮膚を、刺手を用いて1本の鍼管で叩くか（扣管）、両手を用いて2本の鍼管で叩くか（撥指管）の違いであり、目的と作用はほぼ同じです。

● 撥指管・遠覚管

遠覚管も、2本の鍼管を用いて刺針部位の周囲の皮膚を叩くという技法は撥指管と共通していますが、抜針した後に叩くというところが異なります。

また、扣管と撥指管が補法にも瀉法にも用いられるのに対し、遠覚管は抜針した針痕を閉じずに針痕周辺の邪気を発散させ、筋緊張をゆるめるという明確な瀉法の目的で用いられます。

◎ 扣管（こうかん）　Tapping around Kan

● 名称の由来

「扣」は「叩く」という意味で、この術は、撥指管と同様に、1本の鍼管で皮膚をはじくようにリズミカルに叩くことから、この術は扣管と名付けられた。

● 主な作用

表層に鬱滞した邪気を発散して疼痛を軽減する（瀉法）。

● 鍼管の持ち方

刺手の示指を管頭に当て、母指と中指と薬指で鍼管を縦に持ち、小指を薬指に添わせる。

扣管

<ruby>扣管<rt>こうかん</rt></ruby>

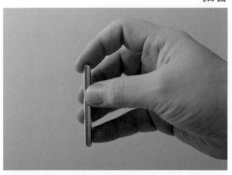

【持ち方】 示指頭を管頭に当て、母指と中指・薬指とで管を挟み、小指は薬指に添える。

①針を刺入したら、押手を離す。
②刺手で管を持ち、管先で皮膚を細かく叩く。
③また違う方向から、
④管先で皮膚を細かく叩く。
⑤また違う方向から、
⑥管先で皮膚を細かく叩く。
⑦このように周囲から、
⑧管先で皮膚を細かく叩く。

● **技法**

針を目標とする深度まで刺入し、刺手と押手を針から離し、刺手の示指を管頭に当て、母指と中指と薬指で鍼管を縦に持ち、小指を薬指に添わせ、刺入された針の周囲を連続的に叩く。

四肢の末端の経穴など、浅くしか刺針ができない場合には、刺針した針体の針柄を押手で軽く把握し、針の周囲を叩く。

● **使用例**

歯の痛みや偏頭痛で側頭部に邪熱がある場合に、角孫穴に横刺で刺針した後に扣管を用いることで、筋緊張をゆるめ、側頭部の痛みを緩和する（瀉法）。

風邪をひき悪風する場合、大杼穴に刺針した上で、項や肩甲間部に扣管を用いることで、腠理を開き、発汗を促すことができる（瀉法）。

膝が曲がり筋肉が緊張している場合に、懸鐘に上方に向けて刺針し、この術を用いて下腿外側の筋肉をゆるめる（補法）。

下腹部が脹満する場合に、下腹部を補った上で、内庭と公孫に用いる（誘導）。

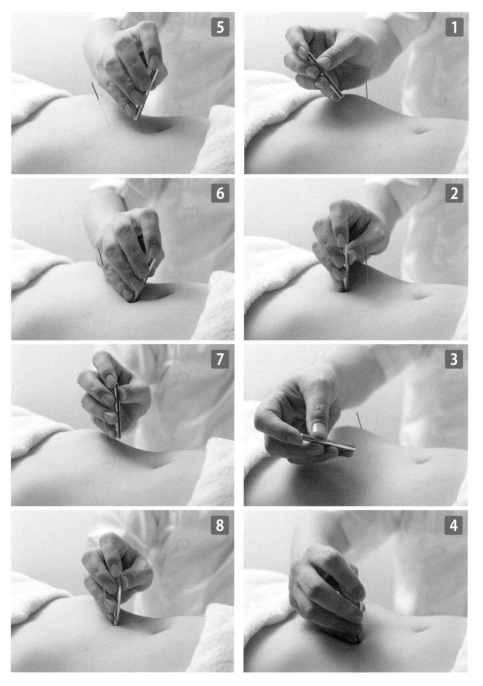

◎撥指管　Spring finger Kan
(はっしかん)

●名称の由来

「撥」は「はじく」という意味で、この術は、両手の指で鍼管を持ち、皮膚をはじくようにリズミカルに叩くことから、この術は撥指管と名付けられた。

●主な作用

気滞や熱邪を発散させる（瀉法）。

気血を巡らせる（補法）。

●鍼管の持ち方

両手の示指を管頭に当て、母指と中指と薬指で鍼管を縦に持ち、小指を薬指に添わせる。

●技法

針を目標とする深度まで刺入し、刺手と押手を針から離し、両手で鍼管を縦に持ち、2本の管先で刺入された針の周囲の皮膚を、軽くリズミカルにまんべんなく叩く。叩く回数は多いほど良い。扣管と同様の術を、両手を用いて行うことで、さらに細かくリズミカルに刺激する術である。

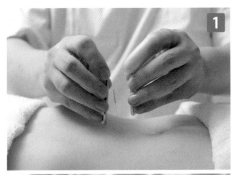

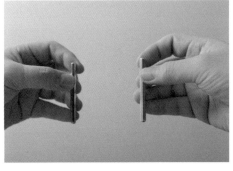

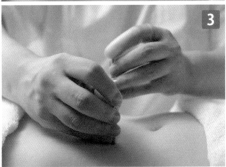

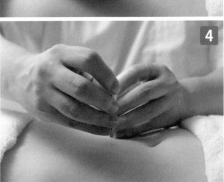

【持ち方】　両手の示指頭を管頭に当て、母指と中指・薬指とで管を挟み、小指は薬指に添える。

①両手に鍼管を持ち、右手の管先で皮膚を叩き、
②左手の管先で皮膚を叩き、交互にくり返し叩く。
③また違う方向から同様に、右手の管先で皮膚を叩き、
④左手の管先で皮膚を叩く。周囲から交互にリズミカルに叩く。

● 使用例

胸中が息苦しい場合に、膻中や中府に用いる（瀉法）。

足が冷えて痺れ、動かしにくい場合に、承山に用いる（補法）。

子宮からの不正出血に対して、陰谷、照海、然谷のいずれかに扣管を用い、懸鐘に撥指管を用いる（誘導）。

◎遠覚管　Far sense Kan
（えんかくかん）

●名称の由来
針を抜いた後に、刺針部位より遠く周囲にまで、瀉法の効果を広げることを目的として、両手で鍼管を持ち皮膚を叩くことから、この術は遠覚管と名付けられた。

●主な作用
虚実寒熱にかかわらず、疼痛全般に用いる（瀉法＋補法）。
鍼痕周辺の邪気を発散し、筋緊張をゆるめる（瀉法＋補法）。

●鍼管の持ち方
撥指管と同様に、両手の示指を管頭に当て、母指と中指と薬指で鍼管を縦に持つ。

●技法
遠覚管は、抜針後の処置法である。目的の深さまで刺入して瀉法を行い、針を抜いた後に、両手で鍼管を縦に持ち、管先を皮膚に当てて、抜針した周囲の皮膚をリズミカルに叩く。

遠^{えん}覚^{かく}管^{かん}

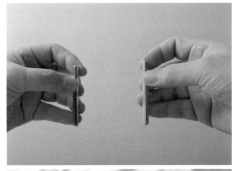

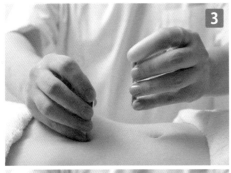

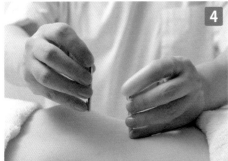

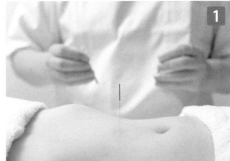

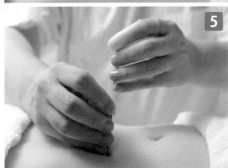

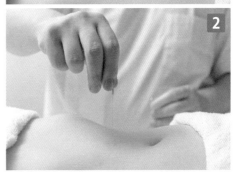

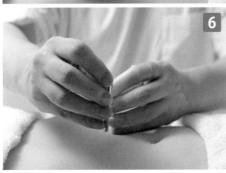

【持ち方】　両手の示指頭を管頭に当て、母指と中指・薬指とで管を挟み、小指は薬指に添える。

①補瀉を施し終えたら、
②針を抜き去り、
③両手に鍼管を持ち、右手の管先で皮膚を叩き、
④左手の管先で皮膚を叩き、交互にくり返し叩く。
⑤また違う方向から同様に、右手の管先で皮膚を叩き、
⑥左手の管先で皮膚を叩く。周囲から交互にリズミカルに叩く。

● 使用例

足関節の腱が引きつれて骨が痛む場合に、商丘と照海に用いる（瀉法）。

◎随肉管（ずいにくかん） Muscle rubbing Kan

● 名称の由来

「肉を随える管」という意味。気血を集めることを目的として、鍼管で刺針部位の周囲の筋肉を摩擦することから、この術は随肉管と名付けられた。

● 主な作用

気血が虚して冷えた患部に気血を巡らせる（補法）。

● 鍼管の持ち方

扣管と同様に、刺手の示指を管頭に当て、母指と中指と薬指で鍼管を縦に持ち、小指を薬指に添わせる。

● 技法

目的とする深度まで刺針したら、押手の母指と示指で針柄（竜頭）をつまみ持ち、刺手で鍼管を縦に持ち、その鍼管で針体をまとうように摩擦したり、管先で周囲の皮膚を推し付け肌肉をまとうように摩擦する。

<ruby>随肉管<rt>ずいにくかん</rt></ruby>

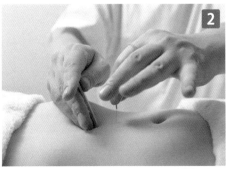

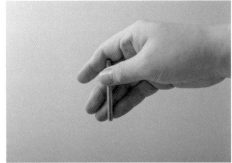

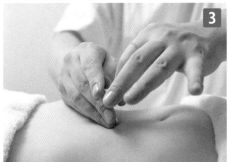

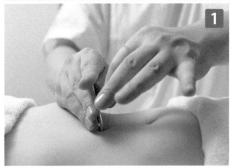

【持ち方】　示指の近位指節間関節横紋に管頭を当て、母指と中指・薬指とで管を挟み、小指は薬指に添える。

①押手の母指と示指で針柄をつまみ、刺手で管を縦に持ち、針体をまとうように摩擦する。
②針の周囲に管先を皮膚に推し付け、
③肌肉をまとうように摩擦する。
④また違う方向から、管先を皮膚に推し付け、
⑤肌肉をまとうように摩擦する。

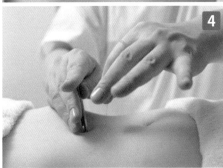

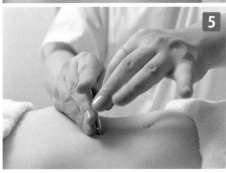

●使用例

冷えによる男子の腹痛、女子の瘀血や気滞による下腹部痛、白帯に対して、腹部に用いる（補法）。

上肢が麻痺して感覚がない場合に、外関に用いる（補法）。

◆④針を振動させる術

竜頭管、巧指管、燃鍼管、内調管、通谷管

【主な作用】

刺針による「響き」「補法」「瀉法」「誘導」の作用を必要に応じて「増強」させ、また、響きと刺激を周囲に「伝播」させます。

気を至らせた後に、穏やかな響きを与えて気血を「調和」させます。

【臨床応用】

浮腫や瘀血や虚証で冷えのある場合には、気血の巡りが悪く、「響き」を得るまでに時間がかかります。そんな場合に、刺針した針に振動を加えることにより、「響き」を早め、「補法」「瀉法」の作用を増強させるために用います。

また、「補法」「瀉法」を施した後、振動を与えることにより、気血の「調和」をはかることができます。

【術の分類】

①針柄を横に振動させる術……竜頭管、巧指管、攙鍼管
②押手のつまみ口を管で叩いて振動させる術……内調管、通谷管

【共通性と相違点】

●竜頭管・巧指管・攙鍼管

竜頭管と巧指管は同類の術です。両者の違いは、刺手を用いて1本の鍼管で叩くか（竜頭管）、両手を用いて2本の鍼管で叩くか（巧指管）の違いであり、目的と作用はほぼ同じです。また、攙鍼管は針を揺らして振動させる術で、目的と作用は竜頭管と巧指管と同様です。

●内調管・通谷管

内調管と通谷管は同類の術であり、両者の違いは、押手を皮膚から離すことなく、針体をつまんでいる母指と示指の爪を叩くか（内調管）、押手を針柄（竜頭）に持ち替え、そのつまみ口を叩くか（通谷管）の違いです。
また、内調管では深い部位に刺入する場合が多く、浅い層から深い層へと2〜3段階で術式を行います。

◎ 竜頭管　Dragon's Head Kan

りゅうずかん

● 名称の由来

鍼管で針の針柄（竜頭）を横から叩いて針を振動させることから、この術は竜頭管と名付けられた。

● 主な作用

響きを促して気を至らせる（響き）。

経絡の末端に気を誘導する（誘導）。

● 鍼管の持ち方

刺手の母指と示指の2本の指で針頭をつまみ、鍼管を横に持つ。

● 技法

針を目標とする深度まで刺入し、刺手と押手を針から離し、刺手の母指と示指で鍼管を持ち、刺入された針の針柄（竜頭）の側面を叩いて針を振動させる。

刺針深度が浅い場合は、針体から押手を離さずに母指頭と示指頭のつまむ力をゆるめた上で、針柄を叩く。

竜頭管
りゅう ず かん

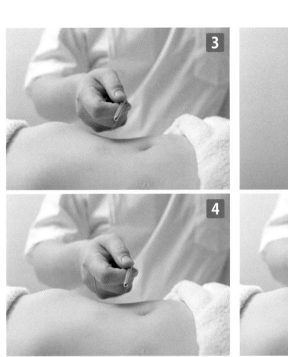

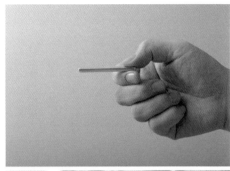

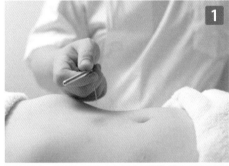

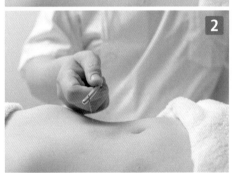

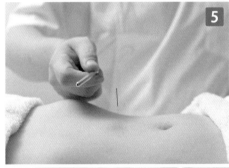

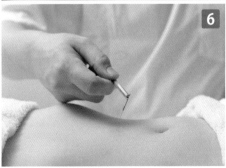

【持ち方】　母指と示指で管頭をつまみ、鍼管を水平に持つ。

①針を刺入したら押手を離し、刺手に鍼管を水平に持つ。
②立っている針柄を右から叩く。
③叩かれた針は振り子のように左右に震える。
④今度は左から針柄を叩く。
⑤同様に針は左右に震える。
⑥また同様に何度も針柄を叩き、針を震わす。

● 使用例

脾胃が虚して脇が引きつれる虚証の浮腫で、胸や脇が痛む場合に、章門（響き）や内関（誘導）に用いる。

手首が腫れて強張る場合に、大陵に用いる（調和）。

手掌が鬱血して熱感がある場合に、内関に用いる（誘導）。

咽喉が腫れて痛む場合に、温溜に用いる（誘導）。

水瀉性の下痢に対して、腹部を温補した上で、復溜に用いる（調和）。

◎ 巧指管 Ingenious Dragon's Head Kan
こう　し　かん

● 名称の由来

両手で鍼管を持ち、鍼管で針の竜頭（針柄）を、横から「巧み」に叩いて針を振動させることから、この術は巧指管と名付けられた。

● 主な作用

響きを促して気を至らせる（響き）。

補瀉法を行い気を至らせた後に気血を調える（調和）。

巧指管

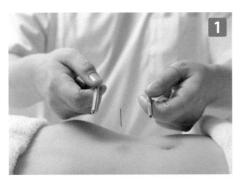

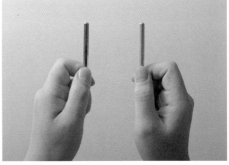

【持ち方】　両手に2本の鍼管を持つ。持ち方は竜頭管と同様に、母指と示指とで管頭をつまむ。

①針を刺入したら押手を離し、2本の鍼管を両手に持つ。
②立っている針柄の右側を、右手の管先で叩く。
③今度は針柄の左側を、左手の管先で叩く。
④さらにまた針柄を右手の管先で叩く。このように左右交互にリズミカルに針柄を叩き震わす。

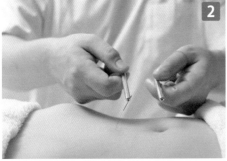

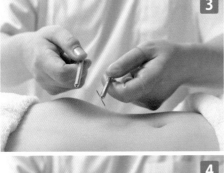

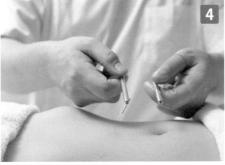

● 鍼管の持ち方

両手の母指と示指の2本の指で管頭をつまみ、鍼管を横に持つ。

● 技法

針を目標とする深度まで刺入し、刺手と押手を針から離して両手の母指と示指で2本の鍼管を持ち、刺入された針の針柄（竜頭）の左右の側面を叩いて針を振動させる。竜頭管と同様の術を、両手を用いて行うことで、さらに細かくリズミカルに刺激する術である。

● 使用例

肘の筋肉が引きつり骨の付着部の腱が痛む場合に、曲沢と尺沢と曲池に用いる（調和）。

膝から股関節にかけて痛む場合に、風市に用いる（調和）。

◎ 熿鍼管　こうしんかん　Glowing Needle Kan

● 名称の由来

「熿」は光り輝く意味。鍼管で針を振動させることで、針が輝いて見えることから、この術は熿鍼管と名付けられた。

こうしんかん
熯鍼管

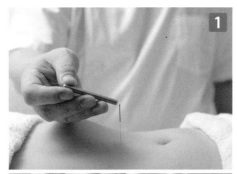

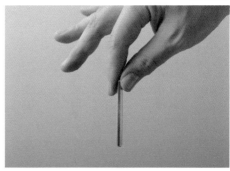

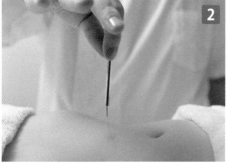

【持ち方】　母指と示指の先端で管頭を軽くつまみ、鍼管を縦にぶら下げる。

①刺入した針の針柄頭から、管先をはめる。
②針柄の半分ほどまで管先をはめた状態。
③振り子を振るように、管先と針柄を左に振り、
④今度は右に振る。左右に連続的に管先と針柄を振る。

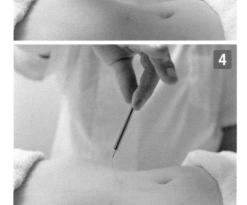

● 主な作用

響きを促して気を至らせる（響き）。

周囲に軽い響きを伝える（響き）。

● 鍼管の持ち方

刺し手の母指と示指の2本の指で、鍼管の上部をつまむようにして持つ。

●技法

針を半分過ぎまで刺入したら、押手を離し、針柄（竜頭）の半分まで鍼管を入れ、刺し手の母指と示指で鍼管の上部をつまみ、振り子のように鍼管と針を振動させる。

●使用例

足が腫れて痛む場合に、膝眼に用いる（響き）。

長引く風邪や体力の消耗による慢性的な咳に対して、三焦兪に用いる（瀉法＋補法）。

◎内調管　Internal tuning Kan
（だいちょうかん）

●名称の由来

浅い層から深い層へと2〜3段階に針を刺入するたびに、鍼管で針を叩いて振動させ、体の内部（腠理、血脈、筋骨）を調えることから、この術は内調管と名付けられた。

●主な作用

腹部の気滞、食滞、水滞、血滞を発散させる（瀉法）。

経絡の末端に気を誘導する（誘導）。

内調管
<ruby>内調管<rt>だいちょうかん</rt></ruby>

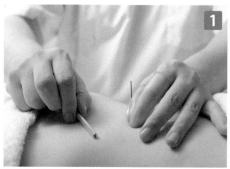

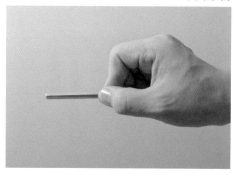

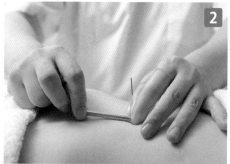

【持ち方】　母指と示指で管頭をゆるくつまみ、鍼管を水平に持つ。

①針を約5mm刺入したら、押手は刺入した針をつまみ、刺手に鍼管を持つ。
②押手の針をつまんだ母指と示指の爪に、鍼管を水平に叩きつける。
③刺手の鍼管を離し、
④また再び押手の針をつまんだ爪に、鍼管をくり返し叩きつける。その後、また針を約5mm刺入したら、同様に叩きつける。さらに針を約5mm刺入したら、また同様に叩きつける。針を引く際も、約5mmずつ段階的に引き、同様に叩きつける。

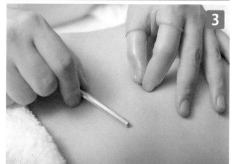

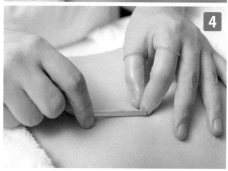

● 鍼管の持ち方

刺手の母指と示指の2本の指で管頭をゆるくつまみ、鍼管を横に持つ。

● 技法

針を直刺で三、四分（約10ミリ）刺入したら、針をつまんでいる押手の母指と示指の爪を鍼管で叩く。針を震わせ針先に振動を伝えるためである。同様にして中間層、深い層へと度々刺入しては、押手の母指と示指の爪を叩く。抜針する時も、三、四分ずつ引いては、押手の爪を叩く。

内調管は、主として腹部など、針を深く刺入することが可能な部位に用いられ、四肢の経穴などに用いる場合には、浅く2段階に刺入して用いる。

● 使用例

上腹部の水滞によるしゃっくりに対して、中脘に用いて水滞を発散し、同時に上腹部や心下部の気血を巡らせる（瀉法）。

便と気（ガス）が停滞して下腹部が痛む場合に、帰来に用いて便通を促し痛みを軽減する（瀉法）。

関節の疼痛に対して、合谷、足三里、委中、陽池、大杼に浅く2段階に刺入して用いる（瀉法）。

風邪による頭痛、発熱に対して、腹部を補い、頚部を瀉した後、委中に用いて上部の実熱を下に誘導して調える（誘導）。

便秘に対して、下腹部に刺針した後、足三里に用いて便を下に引き下ろす（誘導）。

◎通谷管(つうこくかん)　Connecting valley Kan

●名称の由来

「谷」は「陥凹部」という意味で、骨間の谷間（関節の陥凹部）に気を通すことを目的として用いられることから、この術は通谷管と名付けられた。

●主な作用

気血の虚損による足や膝の関節の疼痛に対し、疼痛の部位の周囲に用いて気血を導く（補法）。

●鍼管の持ち方

刺手の母指と示指の2本の指で管頭をゆるくつまみ、鍼管を横に持つ。

●技法

針を目的とする深度まで刺入したら、押手の母指と示指で針柄（竜頭）をつまみ、その押手のつまみ口と針柄との間を、刺手の母指と示指で持った鍼管の先端部分で、押手の母指を滑らすようにして連続的に叩く。

●使用例

足の筋肉が引きつり痛む場合に、足の三隅穴（解渓・地五会・申脈）に用いる（補法）。

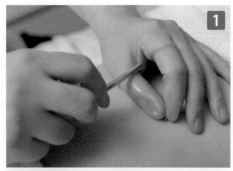

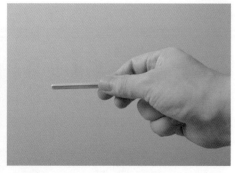

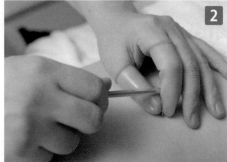

【持ち方】 母指と示指で管頭をつまみ、鍼管を水平に持つ。

①針を目的の深さまで刺入したら、押手の母指と示指で針柄をつまみ、刺手は鍼管を持つ。
②管先で押手の母指を滑らすようにして、押手でつまんだ針柄に管先を叩きつける。
③また刺手の鍼管を離し、
④同様に針柄に管先を叩きつける。連続して叩きつけ、針を振動させる。

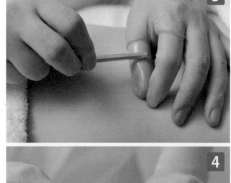

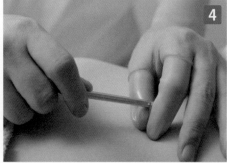

発熱、悪寒する場合に、大椎周囲に浅く刺針し、この術を用いて発汗を促す（補法）。

Chapter 6

管鍼法の創案者・杉山和一

◆日本鍼灸の父

もし、あなたが、鍼の臨床に「鍼管」を使用しているとしたら、杉山和一の名を知っておくことが必要です。

なぜなら、鍼の施術に鍼管を使用する「管鍼法」は、17世紀の日本において杉山和一によって確立され、日本全土に広められたからです。そして、現在では、管鍼法は刺針法の世界標準となりつつあります。

そのため、杉山和一は、管鍼法を確立し、広めたことで、鍼灸史上で最も偉大な鍼医として認められており、また日本では、徳川幕府の五代将軍徳川綱吉の侍医であったことでも知られています。そして、海外においても、Waichi Sugiyama の名は、「日本の鍼の父」(The father of Japanese acupuncture) として鍼灸師たちの尊敬の念を集めています。

杉山和一は400年以上も前に誕生した人物であるため、現在においては不明なことや不確実なことも少なくありません。そこで本書では、できる限り史実に近い話として、杉山和一についてご紹介したいと思います。

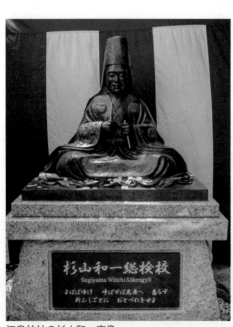

江島神社の杉山和一座像

92

◆盲目となり鍼医を志す

杉山和一は、1610（慶長15）年に、伊勢国（今の三重県）の津で、杉山重政という200石取りの中級武士の長男として生まれました。時は、戦国時代が終わり、1600年に関ヶ原の合戦があって、1603年に徳川家康が江戸に幕府を開いて間もない頃です。

彼は健康な体で生まれましたが、幼少期に、はしかと推測される伝染病に感染したことが原因で視力を失いました。彼が失明した歳は、5歳という説と10歳という説があります。

この時代、視覚障害者の職業は、琵琶法師か「揉み療治」と呼ばれる按摩というのが一般的でした。そのため、和一の母は彼に琵琶を習わせましたが、彼は琵琶法師になることを望みませんでした。

16歳となったある日、和一は、自分が琵琶法師ではなく鍼医を志したいと両親に告げました。彼は心の優しい性格であり、まだ目が見えていた幼い頃は、殺し合いをする武士ではなく人を助ける医者になりたいと考えていたのです。

当時、鍼医を目指すということは並大抵のことではありませんでした。ましてや、視覚障害者にとっては、よほどの覚悟がなければ成し遂げられることではありません。実際に当時、視覚障害者の鍼医は日本全国でも三人しかいませんでした（山瀬琢一、山川城官、岩船城泉）。

つまり、視覚障害者が鍼医になるというのは、限りなく不可能に近い目標であったのです。しかし、和一の決心は固く、父親の重政も、彼の志を理解して支持することを決めました。

この時代、鍼を学ぶためには、京か江戸まで行かなくてはなりませんでした。また、視覚障害者は視覚障害者から学ぶのが慣例でしたが、和一が暮らす伊勢国により近い京には、盲目の鍼医はいませんでした。そして、彼らは、江戸に山瀬琢一という盲目の鍼医がいることを知り、重政は彼を探し当てました。

重政は琢一に、和一を弟子にしていただけるようにお願いする手紙を書き、琢一は最終的にそれを承諾しました。そして、1626（寛永3）年、和一が17歳の時、彼は下男を伴って江戸に渡りました。

山瀬琢一は、最初から和一に鍼術を教えたのではなく、最初の約3年間（1626～1630年）はもっぱら「按摩」を教えました。

視覚障害者が鍼術を行うためには、視覚以外の感覚によって人間の体を深く知ることが不可欠となります。そのため、手で触れることによって人の体を理解できるようにするために、琢一はまず揉み療治を和一に教えたのです。

そして、和一は熱心に揉み療治の修行を積み重ね、その技術は順調に上達しました。

琢一に入門して約3年が過ぎ、和一が揉み療治の技術を全て習得すると、琢一は和一に鍼術を教え始めました。しかし、ここで和一は致命的な不測の事態に直面することになり、そのことで、彼は鍼術の修行を続けることができなくなってしまいます。

一説には、和一は愚鈍で怠惰であったために、鍼の技術を習得できず、山瀬琢一から破門されたと伝えられています。しかし、和一が破門になった本当の理由を知るためには、当時の鍼術に関する時代背景を知ることが不可欠です。

当時の日本の鍼術の世界には満足な教科書などは存在せず、鍼治は、ごく簡単な穴法図に基づき、師匠の口

述による指導によってのみ行われていました。そのため、当時の鍼治には誤治も多く、誤治によって患者が死に至る場合も少なくありませんでした。

また、視覚障害者であった琢一と和一は、穴法図を見ることさえもできませんでした。

当時の鍼術の刺針法は、中国由来の「撚針法」でした。撚針法は、太くて長い針（推定10番以上）を、母指と示指で捻りながら一気に刺入する刺針法です。この刺針法では、刺針時の刺激が極めて強力であったため、患者が気絶する場合もあり、また、そのまま絶命してしまう場合もありました。

そのため当時は、気絶した患者に対する「返し針」を習得することが必須でした。当時の鍼術には、医療過誤や医療事故がつきものであったということです。

和一は、心の優しい性格であったため、いつか自分も医療事故を起こして、患者を死なせてしまうかもしれないということを、どうしても受け入れることができませんでした。そして、そのことが要因となって、鍼術の修行を続けることができなくなってしまいました。

山瀬琢一に入門して約3年、和一がまだ20歳の時のことです。しかし、和一が撚針法を習得し、修行を前に進めることができなければ、琢一は和一を破門にすることを余儀なくされます。

鍼医の道を志し、そのために、約3年間、熱心に按摩の修行に励んできた弟子を切り捨てるというのは、琢一にとっては断腸の思いであったことでしょう。しかし、最終的に和一は、琢一から破門にされてしまうことになります。

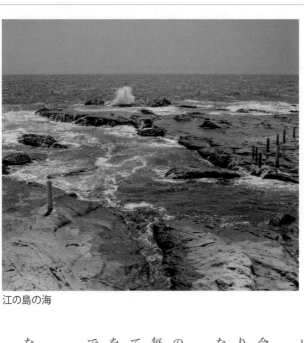
江の島の海

◆挫折を経て御神託を授かる

鍼医の道を諦めるということは、琵琶法師になるか、それとも死ぬかという二つの選択肢しか、和一には残されていないことを意味しています。しかし、和一は、どうしても鍼医の道を捨てることができませんでした。

そこで、この上は、もはや「神仏の力」におすがりするしかないと考え、江の島の弁才天に参詣することを決意しました。

江の島の弁才天は、欽明天皇（510年頃～571年）の勅命により、「御霊窟」と呼ばれた岩屋に宮を建てたのがはじまりとされ、当時は関東地方の最高峰の霊場として崇敬の的となっていました。

江の島の岩屋は、波によって浸食されてできた洞窟です。江の島の弁才天では、「宿坊」と呼ばれる宿泊施設から岩屋まで、毎日通って願をかける「お籠り」と呼ばれる断食修行が行われていました。杉山和一は、「下之坊」と呼ばれる宿坊で寝泊りをしながら、21日間、水以外は口にせず、1日に3回、岩屋まで通って御神託を授かるための断食祈願を行いました。

この断食修行は、水以外は一切口にすることができない過酷な修行であり、当時は、修行中に命を落とす人も少なくありま

96

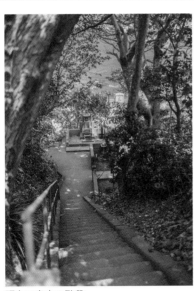

現在の島内の階段

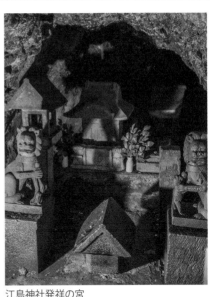

江島神社発祥の宮

せんでした。そのため、神の御神託を授かることができなかった場合には、死ぬ覚悟ができていなければ、このお籠り修行はできません。

つまり、杉山和一は、御神託を得るために、死さえもいとわぬ覚悟で江の島での修行に臨んだということです。

当時、下之坊であった現在の辺津宮から岩屋まで、私も実際に歩いてみました。辺津宮から岩屋まではかなりの距離があり、また、江の島の地形は高低差が激しく、長い階段の上り下りを何度も繰り返さなければ、岩屋にたどり着くことはできません。

現在は、階段や橋が設置されていますが、当時は階段も橋もなく、下男を伴っていたとはいえ、盲目の身で1日3回、下之坊と岩屋を往復したというのは驚異的なことです。おそらく1日がかりであったと考えられます。

杉山和一が命を落としてでも得たかった神の御神託とは、「鍼術による医療事故を防ぐための方法」でした。和一が修行を続けるため、そして鍼術の道が健全に発展していくためには、施術の安全性を確保することが、どうしても必要だったのです。

和一は、清助という下男を連れて江の島の弁才天を訪れ、下

之宮で修行を始めました。当時、江の島の弁才天のお籠り祈願は、7日間をひと区切りとして行われていました。そこで、和一は御神託を授かるために、江の島の下之宮で、飢えと寒さの極限状態の中で7日間にわたって断食祈願を実行しました。

しかし、結果としては、何の御神託も授かることができませんでした。そこで、さらに7日間、断食祈願を続けましたが、やはり、何の御神託も授かることはできませんでした。この修行では、多くの人が10日間ほどで命を落としてしまいますから、14日間の修行で生き残っただけで奇跡的なことです。

しかし、和一は、さらに7日間、断食を続けました。すると、和一の脳裏に、生死をかけて祈念し続けた弁才天が姿を現し、「針をより安全で容易に打つために管のような補助道具を使う」という天来の妙想が閃きました。管鍼法は、和一の命がけのお籠り修行によって、最後の最後に得ることができた御神託だったのです。

講談の「杉山和一苦心の管鍼」では、断食祈願の満願の日、石につまずいて転んだ拍子に木の葉にくるまった松葉が体に触れたことで、鍼管という着想を得たと弁じられていますが、真偽のほどは定かではありません。

いずれにしても、現代において、私たちがごく当たり前のように用いている管鍼法は、鍼術による医療事故の防止を願う一心で、杉山和一が生死を賭けて手に入れた賜物であったということです。

◆京で「管鍼法」を確立する

江の島で弁才天の啓示を得て、断食修行を終えた和一は、江戸の山瀬琢一の元に戻っています。そして、断食修行の成果として、御神託によって「鍼管」という着想を得たことを琢一に報告しました。

和一は、これよりさらに5年間（1630〜1635年）、破門になったはずの琢一のもとで、再び鍼術の修行を積んでいます。おそらく琢一は、和一の管鍼法の構想を理解して支持していたのであろうと考えられます。

こうして5年がたつと、琢一は、和一に江戸を離れて京に行くことを勧めました。当時の日本では、鍼術の本場と言えば京であり、鍼術が江戸よりも盛んに行われていました。そのため、京には優れた鍼医たちが集まっていたばかりでなく、鍼術に関する様々な情報も集まっていました。また、鍼術の道具を作る職人も、江戸より大勢いて、針の製造技術も進んでいました。

京は、神社仏閣が多い土地柄であるため、金属加工自体の技術水準が、他の地域よりも大幅に高かったものと考えられます。そして、こうした針の製造技術や金属の加工技術は、理想的な鍼管や細い針の製造には欠かすことができません。

つまり、和一がさらに鍼術の研鑽を重ね、管鍼法をより高い水準で完成させるためには、京が最適な環境だったのです。そして、山瀬琢一は、鍼術を京の入江流の入江良明に入門して鍼術を学んでいたのでしょう。

このような経緯から琢一は、京に行って「入江流」を学ぶことを和一に勧めました。しかし、琢一の師である入江良明はすでに他界していたため、琢一は息子の豊明に手紙を書いて、和一が彼の元で入江流を学ぶ許可を願いました。

そして和一は、琢一の尽力によって入江豊明から入門を許され、1635年、京へと旅立ちました。

京では実際に、鍼術が江戸よりも盛んに行われていて、入江流の他にも、「御薗流（みその）」「駿河流（するが）」「無分流（むぶん）」「妙（みょう）

針（しん）流」などの流派があり、和一は、入江家の入江豊明のもとで入江流を学びました。

刺針法については、入江流には「図檀掛（ずだんがけ）」と呼ばれる筒（竹筒と推測される）を用いる鍼術の技法が存在していました。そのため、杉山和一が、管を用いて刺針を行った最初の人物ではない可能性が指摘されています。

しかし、杉山和一が金属製の鍼管を発明し、独自の管鍼法を創案して日本全国に広めたというのは明白な事実です。

京には、当時、江戸にはなかった『黄帝内経 素問』『黄帝内経 霊枢』『難経』などの医学書があり、和一は入江家でこれらの書物も学び、1642年までの7年間、入江家で学びました。

そして、入江家で学んだ後、和一はさらに3年間（1642～45年）、京に滞在しています。この間、和一は、妙針流を創始した松沢浄室（まつざわじょうしつ）の弟子の田中知新（たなかちしん）と交流を持ち、また、砭寿軒圭庵（へんじゅけんけいあん）について学ぶなどしたと伝えられています。砭寿軒圭庵は『鍼灸大和文』を著した人物で、「変体仮名書き」というその文体から、おそらく女性であろうと考えられています。

また、京には、御薗流の御薗意斎が創始した「打針術」という独自の刺針法が行われており、入江流では用いられていませんでしたが、京では盛んに用いられていました。打針術は、現在ではおおよそ行われていませんが、小さな木製の槌で針柄の後部を叩いて刺針する鍼術の技法です。「針柄の後部を叩いて切皮する」という独特の手法が、管鍼法の切皮の手法と類似していることから、和一が京で打針術を学び、管鍼法を完成させる上で、打針術が関与している可能性が指摘されています。

こうして、京で過ごしながら、和一は試行錯誤と工夫を積み重ね、「金属製の鍼管」を発明し、「管鍼法」という独自の刺針法を完成させました。

◆鍼術の教科書を編纂

杉山和一が創案した管鍼法は、鍼術において刺鍼を大幅に安全で容易なものにし、切皮時の疼痛を軽減しました。管鍼法は、視覚障害者にとって簡便な刺鍼法となり、日本全土に普及して、現在では刺鍼法の標準となりました。

また、和一は、鍼管を活用して、刺針部位に対して付加的な刺激を与えることを目的とした「十四管術」と呼ばれる技法も創案しました。

さらに管鍼法は、杉山和一が鍼術の歴史に残る「もう一つの偉業」を成し遂げる前提にもなりました。その前提とは、撚針法や打針法では比較的に太い針を使用することが必要であったことに対して、管鍼法は、「極めて細い鍼灸針」の使用を可能にしたということです。

鍼管には一定の内径があるため、刺針時に、針体が鍼管の内径以上にたわむことはありません。そのため、管鍼法を用いることで、極めて細い針を使用しても、針体を曲げることなく円滑な刺針を行うことができます。

そこで、和一は、京で管鍼法に適した細い鍼灸針の開発にも力を注ぎました。鍼管がなければ、細い鍼灸針を使用することもできないことから、細い鍼灸針は、和一の創案した鍼管と管鍼法によって生み出された産物であるといえます。

海外の専門家に、日本の鍼術の特徴は何かと尋ねると、多くの場合、「細い針」「鍼管」という答えが返ってきます。つまり日本の鍼灸の特徴は、江戸時代初期に、杉山和一によってその基礎が築かれたということです。

和一は、ゆくゆくは江戸に戻り、視覚障害者に対する鍼術の教育水準を向上させることで、鍼術を視覚障害

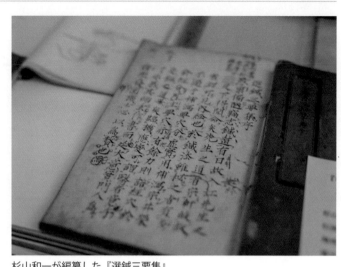

杉山和一が編纂した『選鍼三要集』

者の職業として確立するという目標を立てていました。そのため、京では、鍼管や細い針の開発ばかりでなく、そのための準備も着々と進めていました。

彼は、江戸では学ぶことのできなかった鍼術に関する知識を整理し、鍼術を教えるための教科書の編纂にも着手しました。前述のように、和一が、江戸の山瀬琢一の元で鍼術の修行をしていた頃には、満足な教科書がなかったため、鍼治による医療過誤や医療事故が少なくありませんでした。しかし、それでは、鍼治はいずれ職業として衰退していくことも危惧されるため、杉山和一は修行時代の辛い経験から、鍼術の教育水準を高め、鍼治の安全性を確保することの必要性を誰よりも強く感じていたのでしょう。

そして、心の優しい杉山和一は、自分と同じように鍼医を志す視覚障害者たちに、自分と同じような辛い経験をさせたくないと願っていたのでしょう。

和一が編纂に関与した鍼術の教科書は、『療治之大概集』上・中・下、『選鍼三要集』、『医学節用集』の三部であり、「杉山流三部書」と呼ばれています。これらは鍼治の基礎理論を整理したものです。

最近の調査研究によって、『選鍼三要集』は和一の自著であるが、『療治之大概集』は、和一が京で交流のあった砭寿軒圭庵による、変体仮名書きの『鍼灸大和文』を、漢字・仮名混じり文に再編集したものであること、『医

学節用集』は、和一の死後に彼の講義録を弟子の三島安一が編集したものであることが判明しています。

京での生活が10年を過ぎた頃、入江豊明が亡くなりました。今際の際に呼ばれた和一は、「必ずや、鍼治業道を、後世に至るまで絶えないように努めなさい」と遺言を託されました。

そして和一は、師の遺志を継ぎ、自分自身の目標を実現するために、再び江戸に戻りました。江戸に戻ると、和一は麴町に私塾を開き、弟子を取って開業しました。

鍼術の本場であった京で修行を積んだ和一の鍼の実力により、彼のもとにはたちまち大勢の患者が集まり、その名声によって門弟も大勢集まりました。和一はここで、京で学んだ知識と管鍼法の技術を弟子たちに伝授しました。

この時代、鍼術は家伝のような秘密主義が主流であったことから、私塾を開いて積極的に弟子を取り、自分の技術を公開するというのは非常に画期的なことでした。

◆徳川綱吉の侍医となり、『杉山真伝流』が完成

1670（寛文10）年、杉山和一は、61歳で検校となりました。検校とは、中世・近世日本の盲官（盲人の役職）の最高位の名称です。

杉山和一の鍼医としての名声は、江戸ではさらに広まり、とうとうその名は江戸城にまで及びました。1680（延宝8）年、和一は四代将軍家綱に拝謁し、治療にあたりました。そして、これを機に、和一は江

戸城内においても継続的に治療するようになり、1685（貞享2）年には、五代将軍綱吉の持病を回復させた功績により、常盤門内道三河岸の屋敷を拝領し、以後、将軍付きの侍医とし綱吉に仕えました。綱吉の持病の病名は「ぶらぶら病」であったとされ、それは神経症だとされています。将軍の立場は、極めて強い精神的ストレスを受けることから、おそらく綱吉は何らかのストレス性の症状に悩んでいたのでしょう。

1682（天和2）年、和一の私塾は、徳川幕府から「鍼治学問所」としての認定を受け、1689（元禄2）年には小川町に新規に開設されました。

世界最初の盲学校は、1784年、フランスのヴァランタン・アユイ（Valentin Haüy）らによって、フランスのパリに作られたものとされています。従来は、視覚障害者の教育は個人別に行われていましたが、ヴァランタン・アユイは集団教育へと発展させるためにパリに盲学校を創設したのです。

一方、鍼治学問所は、それより100年も前の1682年に創設されているため、視覚障害者に集団教育を行った世界最初の学校は、実際には杉山和一が創設した鍼治学問所であったということになります。

鍼治学問所は、徳川幕府の支援を得て、幕府より、今後鍼道が絶えることのないよう、鍼治の道を業とする者は、晴眼者と視覚障害者に関わらず、当道座の末々の者に至るまで教育指導することという趣旨のお達しが出されました。当道座とは、860年代に成立した視覚障害者の全国的な互助団体です。

そして幕府は、修行し出精した者を幕府より鍼医として取り立てることを約束しました。

和一は、鍼治の道を志す視覚障害者たちに、鍼治学問所で学び、訓練することを命じ、知識と技術の到達水準によって位を定め、当道座の者は、鍼治学問所の免許を取得しなければ鍼治を行うことができないという規則を定めました。こうして、杉山和一の尽力により、鍼術の教育水準が向上し、施術の安全性が確保され、鍼

治、按摩の道が視覚障害者の職業として確立されました。

鍼治学問所において町の鍼医として育成された杉山和一の弟子たちの中には、幕府や諸藩の医官に登用された者も少なくありません。

杉山和一は、１６９２（元禄5）年5月9日、五代将軍綱吉から、全国の視覚障害者を総督する総検校に任命され、当道座を指揮する立場となりました。

当道座の主な収入の一つには「金貸し」、つまり金融業があり、徳川幕府の保護政策で様々な優遇を受けていました。しかし、その保護政策を逆手に取って、不当な荒稼ぎなどをする者が増え、当道座は、悪徳金融によって次第に腐敗していきました。綱吉はこのような当道座の実情に手を焼いており、当道座の規制を整備し、腐敗を粛清するために、和一を総検校として抜擢したのです。

総検校は、当時の全国の検校の最高の地位として、綱吉が和一に用意した特例的な新しい地位であり、綱吉が和一に対して、鍼医としてばかりでなく自身の参謀としても、その人格と能力に全幅の信頼を置いていたことがうかがわれます。

同年9月29日には、和一は高位の僧官である権大僧都にも任命され、緋衣紋白の裂裟を着用することを認められました。

しかし、これだけの実績を持ちながら、杉山和一は江戸城の奥医師になってはいません。おそらく和一は、「江戸幕府」というよりも「五代将軍綱吉」の個人的な相談役のような存在だったのではないでしょうか。綱吉が46歳、和一が82歳の時のことですから、親子のような信頼関係が築かれていたのかもしれません。

和一は新式目を制定し、大改革を断行して当道座の制度を整備し、当道座を再構築しました。そして、この

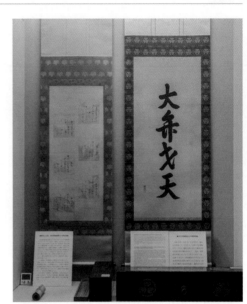
徳川綱吉が本所一ツ目弁天社に贈った直筆の掛け軸

ような和一の功績によって、金融が視覚障害者の健全な仕事として位置付けられるようになりました。

翌年の1693（元禄6）年6月18日、綱吉から、当時の「本所一ツ目」という場所に、2700坪の領地と町屋を与えられました。町屋とは、町人たちが住む土地と家屋のことで、和一は、その家賃も収入として与えられたということです。

さらに綱吉は、老いてもまだ江の島への参拝を続ける和一の体を気遣い、この本所一ツ目の地に、江の島弁才天を一の体を気遣い、この本所一ツ目の地に、江の島弁才天を分霊して祀るよう取り計らいました。そして、このような綱吉の取り計らいにより、杉山和一は江の島弁才天の御分霊をお祀りして「本所一ツ目弁天社」を創建しました。この本所一ツ目弁天社が、現在、東京都墨田区千歳にある「江島杉山神社」です。

1694（元禄7）年5月20日、杉山和一は、一ツ目弁天社の建立を見届けたようにして、この世を去りました。享年85歳。法名は「前総検校即明院殿眼叟元清権大僧都」です。

和一の没後、杉山流は二代目・三島安一の時代になってさらに全国に広まっていき、関東八州中の45カ所に鍼治学問所が開設されました。和一の創案した管鍼法と和一の口伝は、二代目・三島安一、および三代目・島浦和田一によって、流儀書として『杉山真伝流』の名で整理・完成されていきました。

Chapter 7

杉山和一を祀る江島杉山神社

◆江戸の一大名所となる

　杉山和一は、1692（元禄5）年5月9日、五代将軍綱吉から全国の視覚障害者を総督する総検校に任命され、当道座を指揮する立場となりました。そして、1693（元禄6）年6月18日、当時の「本所一ツ目」という土地に、2700坪の領地と町屋を与えられました。

　さらに綱吉は、年老いてもまだ江の島（現在の神奈川県藤沢市江の島）への参詣を続ける和一の体を気遣い、江の島下之宮の祠管を呼び出して、下之宮にあった平家由来の黄金の弁才天尊像を差し出させ、その引き換えとして御朱印地を与えました。

　そして、同日の1693（元禄6）年6月18日、和一に江の島の弁才天尊像を授けて、「江の島への参拝はもう止めるように」との心厚い言葉を賜ったと伝えられています。綱吉の和一に対する信頼と思いやりをうかがい知ることのできる逸話です。

　このような綱吉の取り計らいにより、杉山和一は、江の島弁才天の御分霊をお祀りして「本所一ツ目弁天社」を創建しました。この本所一ツ目弁天社が、現在、東京都墨田区千歳にある「江島杉山神社」です。

　本所一ツ目弁天社は、たちまち江戸庶民の信仰を集めるようになり、「江戸名所図絵」にも掲載されるほどの名所となって、大奥からも舟で参詣に来る人があったと伝えられています。

　和一の没後、弟子たちが、本所一ツ目弁天社に、杉山和一の霊牌所として「即明庵」を建て、和一の尊霊を仏として祀りました。

　1871（明治4）年、当道座が廃止され、一ツ目弁天社は「江島神社」となり、1890（明治23）年、

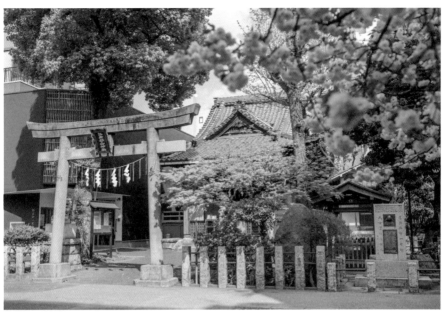

江島杉山神社（東京都墨田区）

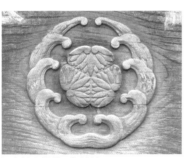

江島杉山神社の御神紋

杉山和一を御祭神とする「杉山神社」が江島神社の境内に創建されました。

1923（大正12）年、関東大震災で二つの社殿が焼失し、その後、第二次世界大戦で再び焼失しました。1952（昭和27）年、社殿が再建され、江島神社が杉山神社を合祀して、社名が「江島杉山神社」となりました。

現在の江島杉山神社では、「市杵島比売命」と「杉山和一」が御祭神としてお祀りされています。また、御賽銭箱と神輿庫の扉に示されているのは、江島杉山神社の御神紋であり、徳川綱吉公に由来する葵が、江の島に由来する波紋の中に表されています。

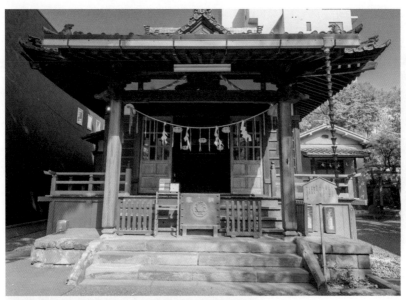

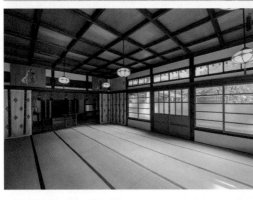

御社殿（外観）
御社殿（内観）

◆江島杉山神社の境内

◎御社殿

第二次世界大戦で焼失した御社殿が、1952（昭和27）年に再建されて、現在の流造の御社殿となり、御祭神を合祀して社名が江島杉山神社となりました。

御祈祷で昇殿する際に拝観できる山本松谷画「一ツ目の弁天」では、1693（元禄6）年の創建当時の面影が残る、明治時代の境内の様子を見ることができます。

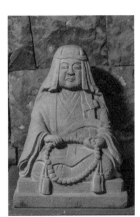

岩屋に奉安された杉山和一の座像

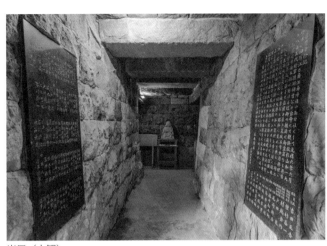

岩屋（内観）

◎岩屋

江島杉山神社の境内には、杉山和一が「お籠り」と呼ばれる断食修行を行い、管鍼法の啓示を授かった江の島弁天の御霊窟を模して1774（安永3）年に築かれた「岩屋」があります。

この岩屋は江の島弁天の御霊窟よりも大幅に小さいもので、内部は丁字路になっています。そして、丁字路の正面の突き当たりには杉山和一の石像がお祀りされており、右手の突き当たりには、「宗像三女神像」、左手の突き当たりには、人頭蛇身の「宇賀神」が祀られています。

この岩屋は1793（寛政5）年10月に修理が行われ、その後の震災では被害はありませんでしたが、1945（昭和20）年3月の戦災による火災で天井の石に亀裂が生じて崩れ落ちたため、旧状を保持したまま鉄筋コンクリートで補強され、山が高くなって現在の外観となりました。

岩屋内では、弁才天のお使いとされる白蛇の形代をお供えすることができます。

◎杉多稲荷神社

神社の境内で、主祭神がお祀りされて
いる本殿とは別にお祀りされている小さ
な神社は「境内社」と呼ばれます。江島
杉山神社の境内には、「杉多稲荷神社」
という境内社が古くからお祀りされてい
ます。創祀年月日と社名の由来はいずれ
も不明です。

◎弁才天と美玉洗

弁天池のほとりに、平成26年12月に完
成した弁天像が奉安されており、その傍らに美玉洗と銭洗が
美玉洗では、江島杉山神社の授与品の「美玉石」を洗うことができます。美玉石、美玉洗の「玉」は、古く
から美しさの象徴とされてきました。参詣に訪れる人々が、水に触れ、祈ることで、美しい福徳の女神である
弁才天の御神徳を賜り、「心身の美しさと若々しさ」というご利益が得られるようにという江島杉山神社の願
いにより、弁天像の傍らに設置されました。
また、銭洗では、硬貨を洗うと金運が上がって富が増えるとされています。

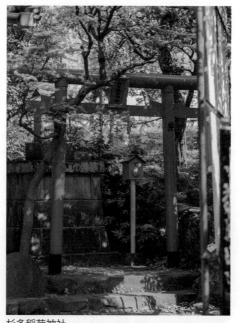

杉多稲荷神社

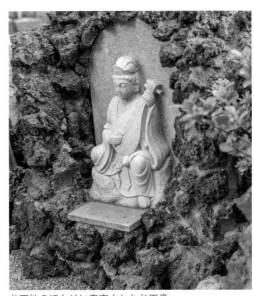

弁天池のほとりに奉安された弁天像

◎即明庵跡の碑

　和一の没後、弟子たちが即明庵を建てて和一の尊霊を仏として祀り、その後、1965（昭和40）年5月18日の和一の命日に、即明庵跡に「即明庵跡の碑」が建立されました。

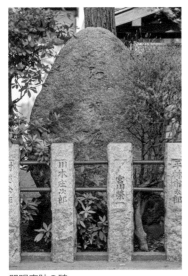

即明庵跡の碑

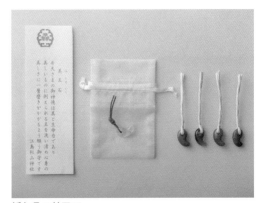

授与品の美玉石

◎ 贈正五位杉山検校頌徳碑

　1924（大正13）年、杉山和一の功績が認められ、正五位が追贈されたのを記念して作製されました。世界で唯一の点字の石碑です。

◎ 力石

　力石は、江戸時代中期より末期まで、庶民の手軽な運動遊戯であった力比べの道具として使われていた大きな石です。

　江島杉山神社がある東京都墨田区内には37個の力石があり、江島杉山神社の境内にある力石は、そのうちで最も重い力石であり、93貫（348・75キロ）の重量があります。

◎ 神輿庫（みこしこ）

　神輿庫には町内の神輿等が保管されていますが、1929（昭和4）年、当時の氏子崇敬者の奉賛により、コンクリート製の神輿庫が建立されました。

　1945（昭和20）年3月10日の東京大空襲によって、境内では本殿が焼失し、岩屋も一部延焼しましたが、この強固

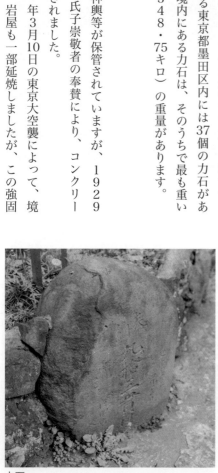

力石

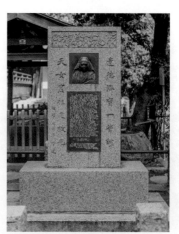

贈正五位杉山検校頌徳碑

な神輿庫だけは焼け残りました。そして、空襲で一帯に火の手が廻る中、当時の宮司家族、近隣の総代等が、弁才天の御神像、綱吉公の掛軸、平家琵琶等を神輿庫に運び込んだことで、それらは火の手を免れることができました。

神輿庫の脇にある「焼け銀杏」も、戦禍で焼けて炭化してしまいましたが、根本から新しい芽が吹き出し、現在でも青々しい葉を茂らせています。

◎平家琵琶「漣漪」

平家琵琶「漣漪（さざなみ）」は山城（京都）の長田左太夫の作で、寛政期（1789〜1801年）に京都の当道職屋敷の二老の職にあった松浦検校・経端一が秘蔵していたものです。

その後、薩摩藩主（島津斉宣または斉興）の手に渡り、江戸の平家宗匠であった麻岡検校・長歳一がこれを賜わりました。

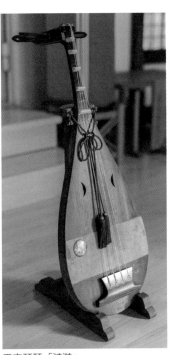

平家琵琶「漣漪」

その後、麻岡検校は弟子の福住順賀一にこの琵琶を与えました。琵琶の収められている箱の蓋裏には、福住が関東の惣録職を無事に勤め上げたことに感謝して、文久2（1862）年に、惣録屋敷にゆかりの深い一ツ目弁才天に奉納したと記載されています。当道座の錚々たる検校たちが秘蔵し、受け継がれてきた名

器であったことが推察されます。

2000（平成12）年と2016（平成28）年の2度の修理が行われ、2000年の修理の際、槽内に1823（文政6）年と1858（安政5）年の2度の修理に関する墨書が認められました（琵琶は製作歴や修理歴を槽内や腹板の裏側に記す習慣があります）。

本所一ツ目の惣録屋敷では、京都の職屋敷に倣い、弁才天社で当道座の二大年中行事である積塔会と涼塔会の儀式が行われており、その儀式の中では、弁才天に平家琵琶の演奏が奉納されていました。その様子は『遊歴雑記』や『東都歳時記』に見ることができます。

◎杉山和一記念館

江島杉山神社の境内の一角には、「杉山和一記念館」があります。この記念館は、「公益財団法人杉山検校遺徳顕彰会」が杉山和一生誕400年を機に「平成の鍼治学問所」として企画し、2016年4月に完成しました。

記念館の2階建ての建物の1階には多目的室、2階には資料室があり、「杉山鍼按治療所」も併設されています。

この資料室には、綱吉公御真筆掛軸「大弁才天」、浄光院様御真筆掛軸「六歌仙」が掲げられており、江戸期以降の文献約400冊、江戸時代の経穴人形、鍼灸の道具類約40点など、杉山和一、鍼灸、按摩に関する数多くの展示物があります。この資料室は、墨田区より、墨田区の文化や産業に関連する文献、資料、道具、製品などのコレクションを展示する「すみだ小さな博物館」にも指定されています。

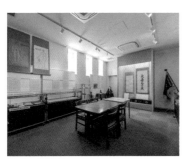

館内の資料室

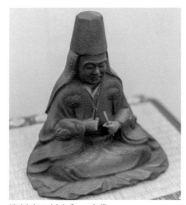

資料室の杉山和一座像

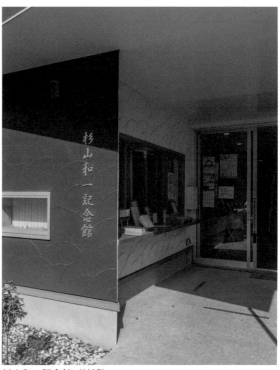

杉山和一記念館（外観）

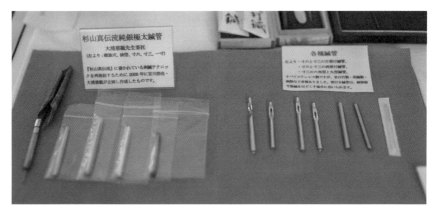

杉山真伝流の純銀極太鍼管（中央より左）と各種鍼管（中央より右）

◆杉山和一と江島杉山神社にまつわる神々

◎市杵島比売命と弁才天

江島杉山神社は、江の島の江島神社の「弁才天」を分霊してお祀りしていますが、御祭神名は「市杵島比売命」です。

市杵島比売命は日本神話に登場する水の女神、海の女神であり、天照大神と須佐之男命が天眞名井で行った誓約によって生まれた三女神の一柱です。『古事記』では「市寸島比売命」と表記されて2番目に生まれた神とされ、『日本書紀』では「市杵嶋姫命」と表記され、その本文では3番目に生まれた神とされています。

天照大神と須佐之男命の誓約では、五男三女神が生まれており、そのうちの田寸津比賣命、多紀理比賣命、市杵島比売命の三女神は、「宗像三神」あるいは「宗像三女神」と呼ばれています。

市杵島比売命は、後の時代の「神仏習合」により、中国から仏教とともに伝来した「弁才天」と習合して同一視されるようになりました。「習合」とは、様々な宗教の神々や教義などの一部が、混同あるいは同一視される現象です。主として、土着の宗教信仰と新しく伝来した宗教が接触し、両者の間に類似した要素がある場合に起こる現象です。

そして「神仏習合」とは、6世紀に日本に仏教が伝来して以降、日本土着の神道と仏教信仰が融合して一つの信仰体系として再構成された宗教現象です。

神仏習合思想には、神道の八百万の神々は、様々な仏・菩薩が衆生を救うために日本の地に現れた権現であ

118

るとする「本地垂迹説」という考え方があります。例えば、八幡神は阿弥陀如来の垂迹、伊勢大神は大日如来の垂迹であるとされました。

神仏習合は言ってみれば、仏教が日本に伝来して興隆を極めた時代に、日本の土着の神々が、外来の仏・菩薩に飲み込まれてしまったような現象であるとも言えるでしょう。そして、神仏習合と本地垂迹説により、市杵島比売命は弁才天と習合して同一視されるようになり、弁才天は神社でも寺院でも祀られるようになりました。

そして、神仏習合の慣習を禁止し、神道と仏教、神と仏、神社と寺院とをはっきり区別させるという明治政府の神仏分離政策により、古くから弁才天を祀っていた神社の多くが、宗像三神か市杵島比売命を御祭神とするようになりました。

◎サラスヴァティー

サラスヴァティー（Sarasvatī）は、肌が白く美しいヒンドゥー教の女神であり、インドで最も古い聖典『リグ・ヴェーダ』によれば、聖なる川の化身とされています。

本来は、水と豊穣の女神ですが、次第に芸術・学問などの知を司る女神としても信仰されるようにもなりました。音楽神、福徳神、学芸神としての側面と鎮護国家の戦勝神としての側面の2面性があるとされ、その像容は、四臂像と八臂像の異なる姿で描かれています。

音楽神、福徳神、学芸神としてのサラスヴァティーは4本の腕を持ち、2本の腕の手には数珠とヴェーダ（ヒンドゥー教とバラモン教の経典）、もう2本の腕の手で「ヴィーナ」と呼ばれる琵琶に似た弦楽器を持っています。

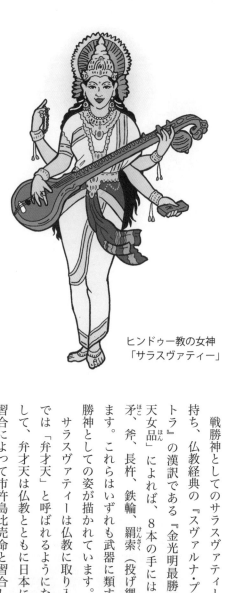

ヒンドゥー教の女神
「サラスヴァティー」

◎弁才天

ヒンドゥー教の女神である「サラスヴァティー」は、中国で仏教に取り込まれ、仏教の守護神である「天部」の一柱として、「弁才天」と呼ばれるようになりました。

8世紀に唐で成立した『大日経疏』(大日経の注釈書)には、サラスヴァティーは「妙音楽天」あるいは「弁才天」であると記載されています。また、仏教教典の『金光明経』では、サラスヴァティー(弁才天)は、智慧、長寿、福徳を与えるとされています。

このように、中国の弁才天はサラスヴァティーのことですから、弁才天と習合した市杵島比売命は、結果的

戦勝神としてのサラスヴァティーは8本の腕を持ち、仏教経典の『スヴァルナ・プラバーサ・スートラ』の漢訳である『金光明最勝王経』「大弁才天女品」によれば、8本の手には、弓、矢、刀、矛、斧、長杵、鉄輪、羂索(投げ縄)を持っています。これらはいずれも武器に類するもので、戦勝神としての姿が描かれています。

サラスヴァティーは仏教に取り入れられ、中国では「弁才天」と呼ばれるようになりました。そして、弁才天は仏教とともに日本に伝来し、神仏習合によって市杵島比売命と習合しました。

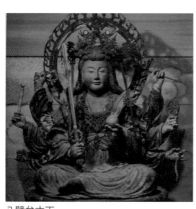

八臂弁才天

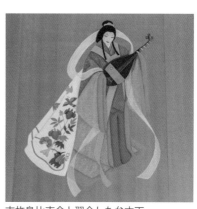

市杵島比売命と習合した弁才天

に、サラスヴァティーと習合したということになります。

中国の弁才天はサラスヴァティーと同様に、音楽神、福徳神、学芸神としての側面と鎮護国家の戦勝神としての側面の2面性を持っています。その像容は4本腕の2本の手で楽器を持つ四臂像（四臂弁才天）と、8本腕の手で武器を持つ戦闘的な八臂像（八臂弁才天）の姿で描かれています。

6世紀に仏教とともに中国から伝来した弁才天は、神仏習合によって日本神話の市杵島比売命と習合し、神社でも寺院でも祀られるようになりました。弁才天が市杵島比売命と習合したのは、ともに美しい女神であり、水の神であったことなどの共通性があったことが理由であろうと推察されます。

弁才天は、日本では独自の変容を遂げ、四臂弁才天は琵琶を持つ2本腕の美しい弁才天となり、「妙音弁才天」とも呼ばれるようになりました。弁才天が琵琶を持っているのは、サラスヴァティーが「ヴィーナ」と呼ばれる琵琶に似た弦楽器を持っていることが理由であろうと推察されます。

鎌倉時代には、弁才天は人頭蛇尾の「宇賀神」と習合し、頭上

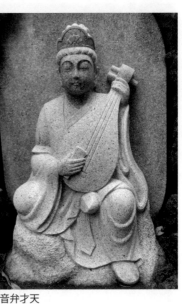
妙音弁才天

『光明経』によれば、弁才天の陀羅尼を唱えれば所願が成就し、財を求めれば多くの財を得ることができるとされています。これが、日本において、弁才天が福徳の女神とみなされる根拠であろうとされています。『金光明経』によれば、弁才天の陀羅尼を唱えれば所願が成就し、財を求めれば多くの財を得ることができるとされています。これが、日本において、弁才天が福徳の女神とみなされる根拠であろうとされています。

鎌倉市の銭洗弁才天宇賀福神社の信仰は代表的で、境内の奥の洞窟の湧き水でお金を洗うと、何倍にもなって返ってくると信じられています。そのため、サラスヴァティーの漢訳は「弁才天」「辨才天」ですが、日本では「弁財天」や「辨財天」と表記される場合もあります。

近世になると、2本腕の弁才天は「七福神」の一柱として宝船に乗り、福をもたらす縁起の良い女神としても知られるようになりました。

日本では、弁才天を本尊、御祭神とする寺社は、「弁天社」と称する場合が多く、江島杉山神社も「本所一ツ目弁天社」と称していました。市杵島比売命が、海の神、水の神であり、サラスヴァティーが、川の神、水

に小さな宇賀神が乗った姿の、「宇賀弁才天」(宇賀神将・宇賀神王)が広く信仰されるようになりました。また、宇賀神との習合により、蛇や龍が弁才天の化身とされるようになりましたが、その所説はインドおよび中国の経典には見られません。

弁才天は、日本では、「弁天」あるいは「弁天様」とも呼ばれ、2本腕の琵琶を持つ弁才天には、財宝神としての信仰が高まっていきました。

の神であることから、弁才天は、海、川、湖などの水が豊富なところに関係するとされ、弁天社の多くが、その近くや島などに祀られました。

そして、弁天信仰が広がるにともない、日本各地で弁才天が祀られるようになりましたが、明治政府の神仏分離政策により、神道色の強かった弁天社の多くは神社となりました。その多くは、宗像三神か市杵島比売命を御祭神とするようになりました。

弁才天を祀る神社では、弁才天の縁日は干支で「巳」の日とされており、60日に一度巡ってくる「己巳」の日は特に縁起の良い日とされています。

◎宇賀神

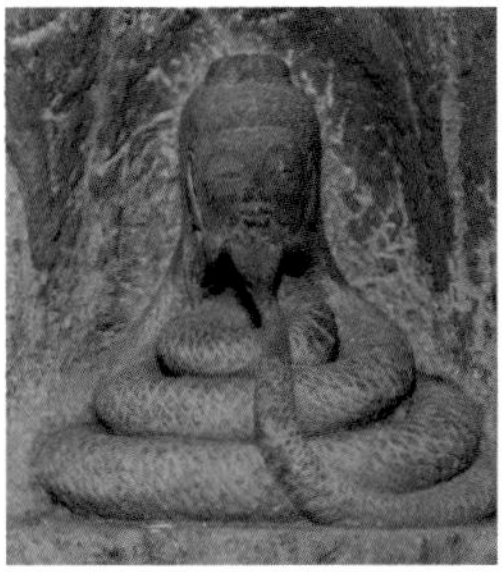

岩屋に奉安された宇賀神像

江島杉山神社の境内の岩屋には宇賀神がお祀りされています。宇賀神は、人面蛇身で蜷局（とぐろ）を巻いた姿の神で、頭部は老翁や女性で一様ではありません。

神名の「宇賀」は、日本神話に登場する宇迦之御魂神（うかのみたま）に由来するという説が有力ですが、出自の詳細は不明です。元々は、宇迦之御魂神と同様に、民間で穀霊神・福徳神として信仰されていた神ではないかと考えられており、また、蛇神・龍神の化身とされる場合もあります。

宇賀神は、比叡山・延暦寺（天台宗）の教学に取り入れられ、弁才天と習合しました。宇賀神と習合した弁才天は、頭上に小さな宇賀神が乗った姿で「宇賀弁才天」とも呼ばれています。杉山和一が深く信仰した江島神社の八臂弁才天も頭上に宇賀神が乗る像容であり、江島杉山神社の岩屋に宇賀神が

123

お祀りされていることに関係しているものと推察されます。

◆江島杉山神社の特徴

◎市杵島比売命と杉山和一

市杵島比売命は、日本神話の美しい水の女神であり、サラスヴァティーは、インド神話の美しい川の女神です。仏教教典の『金光明経』では、弁才天であるサラスヴァティーは、智慧、長寿、福徳を与える女神であるとされています。神仏習合によって習合した市杵島比売命と弁才天は、いずれも美しい女神であり、水の神であったという共通性があります。

一方、医術の神様として江島杉山神社にお祀りされている杉山和一は、徳川五代将軍綱吉公の持病を治して健康管理を任された鍼医であり、生涯現役で、当時としては85歳という驚異的な長寿を生きました。

このように、智慧、長寿、福徳を与える美しい女神である市杵島比売命（弁才天）と長寿の鍼医である杉山和一の二柱をお祀りしている江島杉山神社は、他に例を見ることのない唯一無二の神社であり、数々の御利益があるとされ、崇敬されています。

◎美玉石と美玉洗

江島杉山神社では、「美玉石」という特有の授与品を授与しており、境内の「美玉洗」にて、美玉石を洗うことができます。

硬貨を洗うと金運が上昇して富が増えるとされる「銭洗」は、他の神社にもありますが、「美玉洗」には、美玉石を洗うと身も心も美しく、若々しくいられる御利益があるとされています。美玉石と美玉洗も、他に例を見ることがない江島杉山神社の特徴です。

このように、市杵島比売命（弁才天）と杉山和一の二柱をお祀りして美玉洗のある江島杉山神社は、「健康」「美」「長寿」の御利益がある一大パワースポットとして信仰されています。

「人生百年時代」「長寿社会」といわれる現代社会では、「健康で、若々しく、美しく、長生きをしたい」という人々の願望がますます高まっていることから、大勢の方に御参詣いただき、市杵島比売命（弁才天）と杉山和一の御神徳を授かっていただきたいと思います。

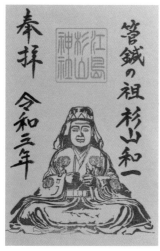

江島杉山神社の御朱印

◎鍼灸師の崇敬神社として

全国の神社については、皇祖天照大御神をお祀りする伊勢の神宮を別格の御存在として、このほかを氏神神社と崇敬神社の二つに大きく分けることができます。

氏神神社とは、自らが居住する地域の氏神様をお祀りする神社であり、この神社の鎮座する周辺の一定地域に居住する方を氏子と称します。

これに対して崇敬神社とは、こうした地縁や血縁的な関係以外で、個人の特別な信仰等により崇敬される神社

江島杉山神社は、前述のような苦心によって、鍼管を創案し、管鍼法を広めた杉山和一が御祭神としてお祀りされている唯一の神社です。

現在では、日本国内のみならず、世界中の多くの鍼灸師が、鍼管と管鍼法の恩恵を被っています。そのため、上記のような神社事情から、江島杉山神社は「鍼灸師の崇敬神社」として、鍼管を用いて臨床を実践する全ての鍼灸師から崇敬されて然るべきでしょう。

そして、実際にも多くの鍼灸関係者と鍼灸師の養成施設の生徒が杉山和一の御神徳を賜り、「鍼治上達」「鍼灸按学術成就」「国試合格」の御利益を得ることを祈願して、江島杉山神社を参詣しています。

江島杉山神社の境内には杉山和一記念館もあり、2階の資料室には、杉山和一、鍼灸、按摩に関する多くの貴重な文献、資料、道具などが展示されています。そのため、鍼灸の関係者の方々には、ぜひ一度は江島杉山神社に御参詣いただき、杉山和一記念館の資料室にも訪れていただきたいと思います。

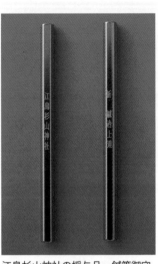

江島杉山神社の授与品、鍼管御守

をいい、こうした神社を信仰する方を崇敬者と呼びます。神社によっては、由緒や地勢的な問題などにより氏子を持たない場合もあり、このため、こうした神社では、神社の維持や教化活動のため、崇敬会などといった組織が設けられています。

氏神神社と崇敬神社の違いとは、以上のようなことであり、一人の方が両者を共に信仰（崇敬）しても差し支えないわけです（神社本庁のウェブサイトより）。

管鍼術の原点・江島神社（藤沢市）

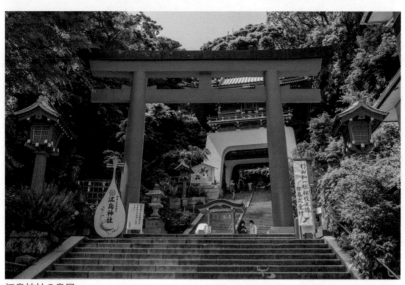
江島神社の鳥居

◆杉山和一が御神託を得た神社

杉山和一が、御神託を得るために断食祈願を行った現在の「江島神社」は、神奈川県藤沢市にあります。

江島神社は、欽明天皇（510年頃〜571年）の勅命により、「御霊窟」と呼ばれた岩屋に宮を建てたのがはじまりとされています。この岩屋は、波によって浸食されてできた洞窟で、現在は、奥行152mと奥行56mの二つの岩屋があります。江戸時代までは「弁才天」がお祀りされており、「江島弁天」「江島明神」と呼ばれて、関東地方の最高峰の霊場として崇敬の的となっていました。

明治政府の神仏分離政策によって、田寸津比賣命を祀る「辺津宮」、「市杵島比売命」を祀る「中津宮」、多紀理比賣命を祀る「奥津宮」の三社からなる「江島神社」となりました。

岩屋に最も近い奥津宮は、昔は「本宮」または「御旅所」と称され、中津宮は昔は「上之宮」と称されていました。辺津宮は、高低差のある江の島の神域内で一番下に位置していることから「下之宮」と呼ばれていました。

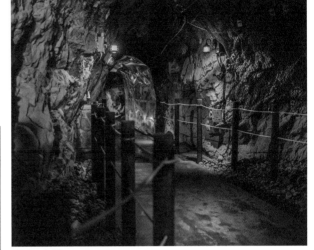

奉安殿に奉安された杉山和一座像

岩屋の内部

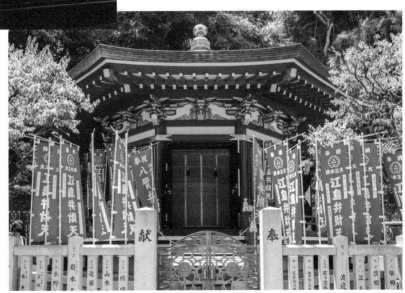

辺津宮境内にある奉安殿

本宮、上之宮、下之宮の三宮には、昔はそれぞれに宿坊と呼ばれる宿泊施設があり、江島神社では毎日、宿坊から岩屋まで通って願をかける「お籠り」と呼ばれる断食修行が行われていました。弘法大師や日蓮も、ここで修行をしたと伝えられています。

杉山和一は、この下之宮の「下之坊」で寝泊まりをしながら、21日間、水以外は口にせず、1日に3回、岩屋まで通って御神託を授かるための断食祈願を行いました。

明治になると、これらの宿坊は宗教と切り離され、一般向けの旅館となりました。こうして誕生した老舗旅館の一つが金亀楼であり、上之坊の跡地に建っていましたが、現在は存在しません。

辺津宮境内の「奉安殿」には、八臂弁才天像、妙音弁才天像、杉山和一木造座像が安置されています。

※本宮の宿坊は、旅館「岩本楼（本館）」として今も存在しています。

◆杉山和一木座像と生誕410年記念像

2020年、杉山和一は生誕410年を迎え、杉山和一と縁の深い江島神社の地元の藤沢市鍼灸・マッサージ師会は、境内に杉山和一の記念像を設置する計画を立てました。

2019年6月、同師会の役員が江島神社に相談に訪れると、相原圀彦宮司が、同神社にも杉山和一縁の像が保管されていることを伝えました。この像は、高さ約50㎝の木造座像で、記念像の製作の参考にするために役員が確認すると、生前に杉山和一本人が作らせた唯一の像であることがわかりました。

この像は、本殿裏の倉庫に安置されていたのか

も不明でした。関係者の間では、鎌倉の一般人家庭にあるという記録を最後に、長らく所在が不明になっていましたが、像の裏に記された「杉山氏　貞享二乙丑年五月十八日」の文字から、行方不明となっていた像であることが判明しました。

また、像本体には損傷もなく、保存状態は極めて良好でした。市や県の歴史博物館の薄井和男館長に鑑定を依頼し、本物という鑑定結果と「仏像彫刻としても一級品。文化財指定にもなり得る」という助言を得たため、修復作業が進められました。

その後、この像は修復作業を終えて江島神社に奉納され、現在は奉安殿に安置されています。

一方、杉山和一の生誕四一〇年の記念像（92頁写真）も無事に完成し、境内の「福石」の傍に設置されました。そして、二〇二〇年九月四日、記念像の奉告祭が行われ、一般に披露されました。

断食祈願の満願の日、和一が福石につまずいた時に管鍼術の妙想が閃いたという伝説が残っており、和一はその後、江戸で開業して出世街道を歩んでいったことから、福石には出世の御利益があると信じられています。

上記のような奇遇ともいえる出来事から、江島神社では現在、杉山和一木造座像と記念像を拝観できるようになりました。

参考
神奈川県全域・東京多摩地域の地域情報紙「タウンニュース藤沢版」
二〇二〇年二月二十八日号、二〇二〇年九月十一日号

本書は、北川毅先生の「日本鍼灸」を海外にも正しく知ってほしいという思いから出発しました。

中国や韓国の鍼灸にはない、気を操る繊細かつ技巧的な日本の鍼灸、その最も特長的な例として私たちは「管鍼法」を取り上げました。

江戸時代に杉山和一が管鍼法を創始したのは、今からおよそ390年前になります。管を使い、細い鍼を用い、正確に穴に痛みなく刺入し、最大限の効果を引き出す。そうした工夫は杉山和一の頃から飛躍的に発展し、現在の日本鍼灸にも引き継がれています。

本書は単なる管鍼法の解説書にとどまらず、日本鍼灸の歴史的背景や文化的特徴にも光をあて、海外の鍼灸医家の皆さんにも理解しやすいように配慮して構成されました。日本人は謙虚さを美徳としますが、自己主張せず海外に正確な情報を発信できないのは欠点でしかありません。本書は勇気をもって、他の国々にはない「日本鍼灸」のすばらしさを主張するものです。

日本鍼灸には多様性と奥深さがあり、杉山流鍼術には「管鍼法」以外にも多彩な手技があります。

本書が、海外の皆さんに日本鍼灸を知っていただく入口になれば嬉しいですし、国内の若手鍼灸師が正しく管鍼法と杉山和一を学ぶ手引書になることを願ってやみません。

本書の執筆に全精力をつぎ込んだ北川先生の英断を讃えるとともに、英訳に当たられたマクギバン美登利先生、出版にご協力いただいたBABジャパンの皆さまに感謝申し上げます。

監修者　大浦　慈観

著者 ◎ 北川 毅　　Author ◎ Takeshi Kitagawa

東京を拠点として世界各地で臨床、教育活動を行う国際派日本人鍼灸師。美容鍼灸の第一人者としても知られている。東洋鍼灸専門学校で特別授業「国際派鍼灸師養成講座」を担当。著書・監修書に、『医学的に正しい美容鍼』『How to 美容鍼灸』（BAB ジャパン）、『おうちで簡単！ お灸エステ』（三栄書房）など多数。

A licensed acupuncturist based in Tokyo, he has been giving lectures in many countries outside of Japan. He is also known as the pioneer and leader in facial cosmetic acupuncture in Japan. He is currently a lecturer at Toyoshinkyu College of Oriental Medicine, and teach the "International Acupuncturist Training" Course. He has written many books including "Medically Correct Method: Facial Cosmetic Acupuncture," "Facial Cosmetic Acupuncture How-tos" (BAB Japan), "At home Quick O-kyu Treatment (San-ei publisher)," etc.

監修者 ◎ 大浦 慈観　　Editorial Supervisor ◎ Jikan Oura

東洋鍼灸専門学校校長。明治国際医療大学大学院鍼灸学修士課程修了。横田観風先生に師事し、日本の伝統的鍼灸および古方漢方を学ぶ。「はり・きゅう治療処路傍庵」院長。杉山検校遺徳顕彰会理事。著書に『腹診による「毒」と「邪気」の診察と鍼灸治療』（ヒューマンワールド）、『DVD BOOK 杉山和一の刺鍼テクニック』（医道の日本社）など多数。

A licensed acupuncturist, and the School Principal at Toyoshinkyu College of Oriental Medicine. After graduating with a Master's Degree from Meiji University of Integrative Medicine, he apprenticed to master Kanpu Yokota and studied Japanese Traditional Shinkyu as well as Ancient Kampo prescription. He has published many books including "Waichi Sugiyama Acupuncture Techniques," "Evil Ki and Poison by Abdominal Diagnosis and Shinkyu Treatment," etc. He is currently a president of an incorporated foundation The Waichi Sugiyama Honoring Association (Kenshokai) and the Director of Shinkyu Hermitage Clinic.

英語共著者 ◎ マクギバン美登利　　English co-author ◎ Dr. Midori McGivern

米国鍼灸専門医／全米ライセンス鍼灸師。外資系マーケティング職で米国や香港駐在後、米国の鍼灸大学院で日本鍼灸を専攻、ニューヨークで鍼灸師として活動。北米東洋医学誌翻訳スタッフ。現在は英国人の夫と共に仏在住、パリ市内で日本鍼灸ベースに診療を行う。

Midori is a doctor of Acupuncture and a National Board-certified Acupuncturist. After working in marketing in the U.S, Hong Kong and Tokyo, she worked as an acupuncturist in NY. Midori currently resides in France and she practices Japanese acupuncture in Paris.

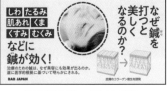
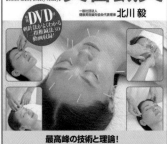
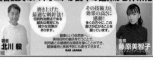

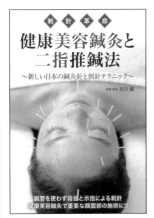
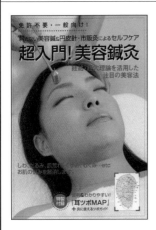
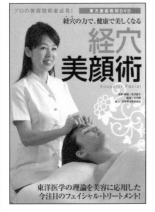

写真撮影 ● 漆戸美保
写真実技 ● 加納覚
イラスト（サラスヴァティー）● 月山きらら
本文デザイン ● 澤川美代子
装丁デザイン ● やなかひでゆき

● 協力 ●
江島神社
江島杉山神社
一般社団法人 藤沢市鍼灸・マッサージ師会
東洋鍼灸専門学校

日本鍼灸の極意 管鍼法
かん　しん　ほう

杉山和一が創案した「十四管術」の実践

2022 年 1 月 5 日　初版第 1 刷発行

著　者　　北川毅
監修者　　大浦慈観
英語共著者　マクギバン美登利
発行者　　東口敏郎
発行所　　株式会社 BAB ジャパン
　　　　　〒 151-0073 東京都渋谷区笹塚 1-30-11　4・5F
　　　　　TEL　03-3469-0135　　　FAX　03-3469-0162
　　　　　URL　http://www.bab.co.jp/
　　　　　E-mail　shop@bab.co.jp
　　　　　郵便振替 00140-7-116767
印刷・製本　中央精版印刷株式会社

ISBN978-4-8142-0429-8 C2047

Kanshin Method

The Essence of Japanese Acupuncture

The Fourteen Kan Jutsu by Waichi Sugiyama

Author: Takeshi Kitagawa

Editorial Supervisor: Jikan Oura

English co-author: Dr. Midori McGivern

BAB JAPAN

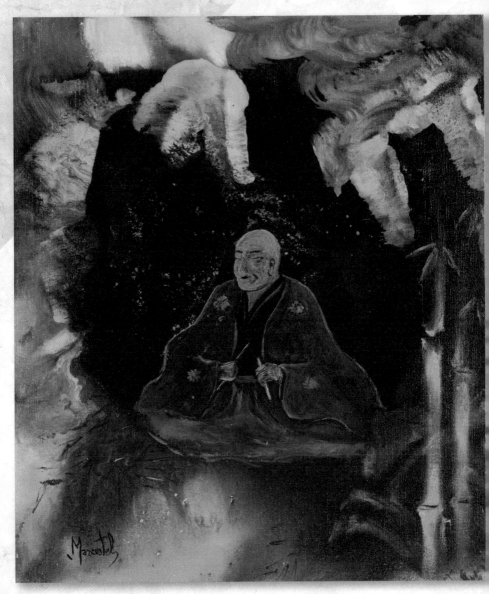

Waichi Sugiyama portrait by Marc Estel

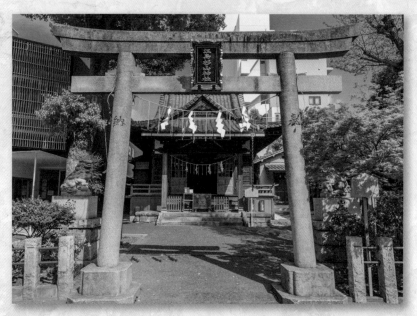

Ejima Sugiyama Shrine (Sumida-ku, Tokyo)

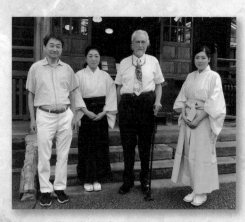

Occasion when Waichi Sugiyama portrait offered to the Shrine in August 2021
(from left, Takeshi Kitagawa, Hiroko Tabe, Marc Estel and Keiko Tabe)

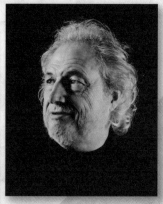

Marc Estel (French artist) is known for his numerous arts connected to ancient Japanese mythology. His arts are available at more than 180 temples and shrines in Japan. In 2014, The Agency for Cultural Affairs of Japan awarded him for "the Bunka Kankeisha Monbukagaku Daijin Award" for his contribution to art and culture.

Since 2010, I have become more involved in Shinkyu clinical and educational activites outside of Japan, both as an educator and an acupuncturist. Experiences working outside of Japan made me think about what is the identity of Japanese Shinkyu? I was often asked what the difference between Japanse Shinkyu is and traditional Chinese Medicine? Also, I noticed most non-Japanese practitioners recognise the usage of Shinkan (guide tube), extremely thin needles are distinctive characteristics of Japanese Shinkyu.

Chinese Medicine arrived in Japan in the 6th century and evolved to become our own- called Japanese Shinkyu. The pivotal point of the Japanese Shinkyu history was in the 18th century, when Waichi Sugiyama invented Shinkan and established the Kanshin Method - an acupuncture jutsu utilizing a guide tube. As using the guide tube became the standard needling method in big countries such as United States, Waichi is now widely known and respected as a father of Japanese acupuncture.

In our modern globalized world, then, how Japanese acupuncturists can answer the question - what is so unique about Japanese acupuncture? In order to answer, or even have a conversation about it, knowing the basics of Waichi Sugiyama is important. You may read a brief summary of his story in Shinkyu educational institutions but is it sufficient to answer above question?

That's the reason we created this book. I thank Mr. Toshiro Higashiguchi, the president of BAB Japan and Mr. Atsushi Moriguchi, the editor of this book for giving us an opportunity to publish such an important book, even making it bilingual so we can spread Japanese Shinkyu to the world. Also, I cannot thank enough Jikan Oura sensei, who is an authority of Kanshin jutsu and Waichi Sugiyama to supervise this book. Equally, Dr. Midori McGivern who worked with me

for a year on the translation, Satoru Kano sensei, as well as both Hiroko and Keiko Tabe, the officials from Ejima Sugiyama Shrine. I am also very proud of my Japanese acupuncturist team who worked with me to create this book together.

*L*ast but not least, while I was writing this book, I encountered a renowned french artist, Mark Estel (Marc Antoine Squarciafichi) who created numerous arts connecting the Japanese spirits and ancient mythology. I was a part of his recovery process from the stroke which left his painting hand paralysed. After his rigorous rehabilitation including Shinkyu treatment, he recovered to create arts again. He recently created a painting of Waichi Sugiyama. His art is now available at the Ejima Sugiyama Shrine.

I feel it's a mysterious coincidence that Marc - a fabulous artist who understands Japanese spirit- regained his health by using Shinkyu and painted Waichi, while I was writing the book about him. Hence, I couldn't resist to show his art in this book. I also encourage you to go and visit the shrine to see the real painting. You might encounter some fortunate event relating to Shinkyu.

Author
Takeshi Kitagawa

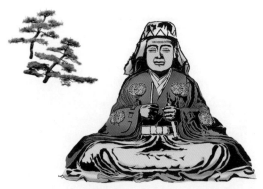

Illustration provider : Ejima Sugiyama Shrine

CONTENTS

Waichi Sugiyama portrait by Marc Estel ...2
Preface...4

Chapter
1

Kanshin Method

9

Chapter
2

Japanese Shinkyu and Kanshin Method

13

Chapter
3

Acupuncture and Ki

29

Chapter
4

Kanshin Needling Method

37

Chapter

5

The Fourteen Kan Jutsu

.... *45*

Chapter

6

Waichi Sugiyama, Founder of "Kanshin Method"

.... *77*

Chapter

7

Waichi Sugiyama's Spirit

.... *91*

Chapter

8

The Birthplace of Kanshin Method

.... *105*

Afterword...110

Chapter 1

Kanshin Method

Kanshin Method and Kanshin Jutsu

Kanshin Method is a unique technique using Shinkan (a guide tube) developed and spread in the seventeenth century by Waichi Sugiyama in Japan.

Kanshin Method is generally recognized as a "needling method using a tube called Shinkan."

In reality, Waichi Sugiyama used the Shinkan not only to insert the needle, but also to give an additional stimulation to the needling point surface skin. He created a variety of techniques called "Kanshin-jutsu," and since the major techniques are counted fourteen, they are called "The Fourteen Kan-jutsu."

Therefore, Kanshin Method needs to be recognized as "the total acupuncture methodology using the Shinkan" including Kanshin-jutsu, rather than considered as just a needling technique. In other words, "needling method using Shinkan" is a narrow sense of Kanshin Method.

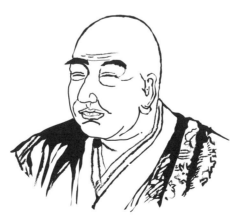

Waichi Sugiyama "the father of Japanese acupuncture"

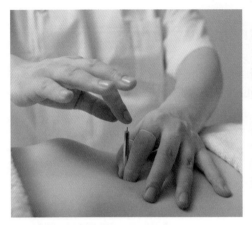

Acupunture with Shinkan "Kanshin Method"

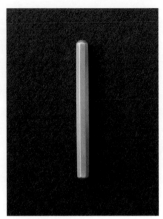

Shinkan (a guide tube)

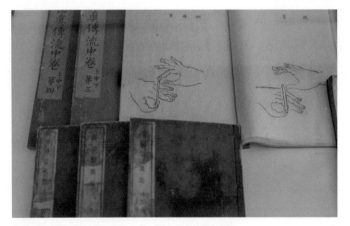

Sugiyama Shin-Den-Ryu ("True-Tradition-School") books

Currently, most Japanese acupuncturists practice needling using the Kanshin method, as this is a standard needling method in Japan. Further, Kanshin method has recently been rapidly spreading globally, many acupuncturists and doctors overseas became familiar with needling using Shinkan. Considering this situation, this book aims to explain more details about Kanshin Method by dividing into the needling method and Kanshin-jutsu for domestic and international doctors and acupuncturists.

English for Kanshin Method

In English, the phrase Kanshin Method is used in a narrow and broad sense. Kanshin Needling Method is used to distinguish as a needling part of Kanshin Method. On the other hand, the Japanese phrase "Kanshin-Jutsu" is used in English for the techniques described earlier.

Kanshin Method:

the total acupuncture methodology using the Shinkan

Kanshin needling method:

a needling method using the Shinkan

Kanshin-Jutsu:

the stimulation methodology using the Shinkan

Chapter 2

Japanese Shinkyu and Kanshin Method

What is Shinkyu?

First, in order to understand Kanshin Method, it is important to be aware what Japanese Shinkyu means. It is much easier if you know a little Japanese language and the background where Kanshin Method was created in Japan, before jumping into the techniques.

First, the word Shinkyu (consisting of two Chinese characters 鍼灸) means "acupuncture and moxibustion." In Japan, most Chinese characters have two different readings and pronunciation. For Shinkyu 鍼灸, the first Chinese character 鍼 is read as "Shin" and it means acupuncture. The second character is read as 灸 kyu, which means moxibustion. For the first character, please note that there are so many other Chinese characters phonetically pronounced as "shin," so phonetically saying shin does not necessarily mean acupuncture. Also, this same Chinese character 鍼 can also be read as "hari," which means needle or acupuncture in Japanese. You can express needle/acupuncture by saying "hari" in Japanese. So sometimes people call Harikyu instead of Shinkyu as "acupuncture and moxibustion." But as Shinkyu is used more commonly among Japanese healthcare workers and acupuncturists, we will call it Shinkyu for this book. The second character 灸 is read as "kyu" and means moxibustion. In Japan, kyu is also called as O-Kyu, as Japanese often add "O" before some words to show respect or politeness (called "honorific prefixes"). As you know, moxibustion is a modality using heat from burning moxa herb which is known for its medicinal values. This Chinese character "灸 kyu," unlike "鍼 shin/hari," is almost always read and pronounced only as kyu (another way of reading is almost never used, so it is not worth mentioned in this book). Please note that people generally refer as "O-kyu," just saying "kyu" verbally may not be understood by Japanese locals ("kyu" phonetically means number 9 in Japanese too).

So, hope it is clear Shinkyu literally means "acupuncture and moxibustion." In Japan and eastern Asian countries, acupuncture or moxibustion can be an independent eastern medicine modality. Each has been known for its medical property and efficacy over a long history. But both share

common characteristics such as using the body's meridian system and acupuncture points, and both have been practiced as a pair in traditional eastern medical treatments for thousands of years. Further, both are known to give safe, effective stimulation to the body to heal from within.

They are almost always used together in Japan, and thus Japanese clinicians do not call "shin/hari" and "O-kyu" separately. Instead they call Shinkyu. On the other hand, in the countries where eastern medicine is relatively new (we are talking about less than a thousand years), such as North America or Europe, acupuncture was well introduced and getting widely used these days. However, moxibustion, or O-kyu, is not very well understood, nor used with acupuncture. The reason could be that acupuncture was first introduced as a single modality to these countries, possibly rather sensationally as an eastern mysterious medicine - no one knew why needling people could be therapeutic at that time. Then moxibustion was less heard of, and less practiced. Further, moxibustion practice might not widely spread as clinical usage of fire is limited or restricted, due to the hospital and clinic environmental regulations in many countries.

As stated, each treatment, acupuncture and moxibustion, has its own method and benefit. Each compensates one another so it is ideal that both modalities are used in one treatment for the patient's benefit. The current situation where acupuncture is considered as a single main modality, and moxibustion has not been recognized as a compatible clinical pair, seems unfortunate in the eyes of practitioners in Japan. We believe moxibustion should earn the same level of recognition and respect as acupuncture has earned, and to be used together, as O-kyu is very beneficial for most patients and clinical cases. In this book, the goal is to introduce Kanshin Method, an innovative needling method which is the most notable characteristic of Japanese acupuncture evolution, and it represents the benefit and superiority of the modern Japanese style acupuncture. But as Kanshin Method is mainly about acupuncture techniques, we do not discuss much about moxibustion in this book. However, acupuncture and moxibustion are both equally respected treatment modalities in east Asia including Japan, and they are greatly compatible to each other, thus should be widely used as a pair. Again, Japanese traditional medicine Shinkyu means both

acupuncture and moxibustion, we want to emphasize this fact before moving on.

We hope we are clear that Shinkyu is different from what is generally practiced in North America or Europe, which often rather focus on acupuncture. For the readers who are practicing or learning eastern medicine outside of Japan, the first take away of this book is perhaps to recognize the Japanese word Shinkyu and its meanings. Further to your recognition, it would be even better if you could remember the word "Harikyu" as well, as explained it is another way to call "acupuncture and moxibustion." Further, there is another little language lesson: as explained earlier, when kyu is used, we explained it's almost always with "O" at the beginning (so people call "O-kyu"), but interestingly, O is not added to the other character "hari" or "shin." Plus, we do not add "O" before Shinkyu either (we never say "O-shinkyu"!). Which words need to add "O" comes with local practice and certain situations, as it involves our historical usage of certain local words. You need to learn each word by heart when you learn Japanese language. Further, the Chinese character 鍼 "hari/shin" is a traditional style Chinese character which is used in Japan. However, in China, simplified Chinese characters are used mostly, and the character 針/针 is the simplified character for needles and acupuncture. So in Japan, you may

---

Our little Japanese lesson clarified below words used in this book :

Shinkyu   : acupuncture & moxibustion

Harikyu   : acupuncture & moxibustion

Hari   : acupuncture

Kyu   : moxibustion

Okyu   : moxibustion(polite form with "O")

also see this Chinese character 針 for needles, such as sewing needles, injections, etc., but eastern medical practitioners in Japan commonly use traditional character 鍼 for acupuncture.

Shinkyu is a Japanese evolution of Chinese medicine which arrived in Japan around 6th century. As it has over 1,500 years of its own history in Japan, it evolved to fit to the Japanese locals. What has been the same is that the acupuncture and moxibustion are always used together to heal diseases and pain. Their fundamental theories and essential usage have been the same as the original adaptation time. However, over the long period of time, Japan evolved to make major differences how to practice them. While Japan was evolving acupuncture and moxibustion locally, a variety of unique acupuncture techniques and tools were developed and shaped the unique Japanese Shinkyu today.

The Uniqueness of Shinkyu

A major turning point of Shinkyu was when Japanese invented Kanshin-Method, extra-thin and disposable needles in the early age while it was shaping its modern development of traditional medicine. These creations represent the uniqueness of Japanese Shinkyu. Besides these, some of the commonly used east medicinal tools - leave-on needles (called "Okibari" in Japanese) such as press needles, also called as press tacks or intradermal needles, as well as some safer or easy-to-use formats of moxibustion including smokeless charcoal moxa or stick-on moxa, etc., are a part of Japanese Shinkyu: they were created in the process of pursuing better, safer and effective treatment for the benefit of both practitioners and patients. These developments represent the Kaizen spirits of Japanese precedent acupuncturists who made relentless efforts to make Japanese Shinkyu more comfortable, effective and safe – the best quality treatment in the world.

clockwise

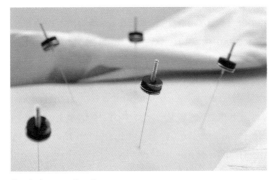

Smokeless moxibustion

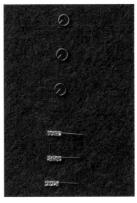

Inter-dermal needles

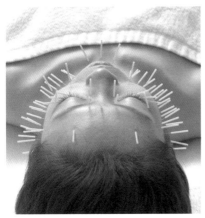

Facial cosmetic Shinkyu (acupuncture & moxibustion)

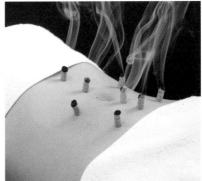

Indirect moxibustion

Superiority and Characteristics of Shinkyu

With its long independent history, what are the major unique attributes of Japanese Shinkyu? Kitagawa, the author of this book has visited many countries, to treat people overseas, as well as to teach Japanese Shinkyu to non-Japanese practitioners in these countries. In many countries, people commented (both practitioners and general public) similar consistent images and perceptions for Japanese Shinkyu as below common characteristics:

- Kanshin-Method (using guide tube) and extra-thin needles
- Sensitive and detailed
- Trusted "Japan-quality"
- Extremely clean and hygienic
- Sophisticated skills and manner

Kanshin-Method and Extra-thin Needles

The Japanese Shinkyu progressed significantly during the seventeenth century. The biggest contribution of the development at that time was the creation of Kanshin-Method using Shinkan (a guide tube), which was newly invented by Waichi Sugiyama. These Shinkan and Kanshin-Method are the main subjects to be introduced in this book. We will get into more detailed techniques later, but around this era in Japan, the major needling method used by many acupuncture doctors was called Nen-Shin-Method which uses much longer and thicker needles around diameter 0.34-1.04mm (gage 28 or less), mostly made of silver or iron . On the other hand, because of the newly created innovative Kanshin-Method, Sugiyama School was able to use much thinner needles, with diameter 0.24-0.32mm. This thinness is still commonly used today, and probably this is the fact that not

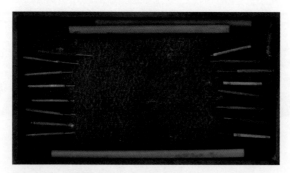

The needles and Shinkan used in the Edo period
(Collection : Satoru Kano)

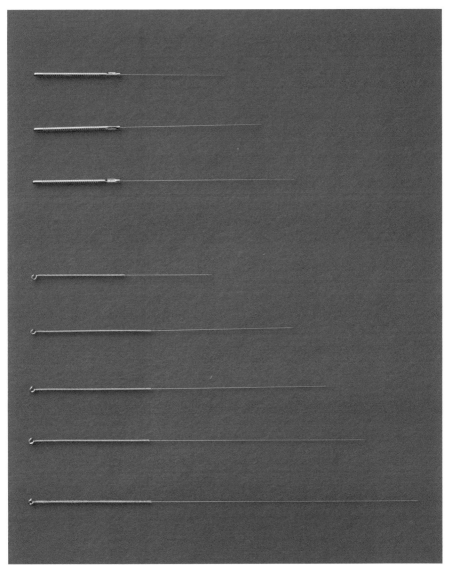

Japanese (above 3) and Chinese (below 5) acupuncture needles (full size)

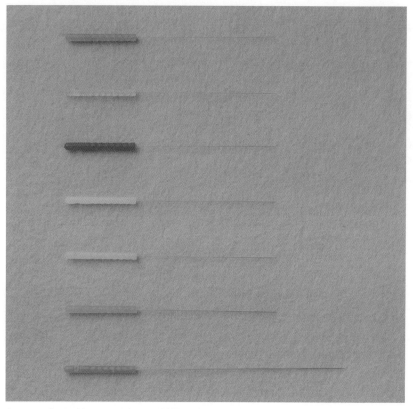

Japanese disposable acupuncture needles (full size)

many people are aware such thin needles were invented such a long time ago in Japan. Then, during the nineteenth century, Japanese refined manufacturing technology to make extra thin acupuncture needles, around 0.10-0.16mm thickness. Again, this thinness is still considered extremely thin as of today, but Japan already had them a long time ago.

Once commonly used needling method Nen-Shin-Method uses thicker needles, and is known to give strong needling stimulation by directly inserting into the skin while the needle is twisted between thumb and index fingers. This method requires higher needle insertion skill, otherwise insertion can be quite painful. Even with the advanced skill, the painless

21

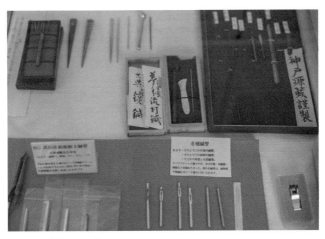

Japanese Shinkyu tools

insertion can be challenging partially due to the thickness of the needles used for Nen-Shin-Method. This insertion method has to use thicker needles, as thinner needles can easily bend on the skin surface when trying to insert. On the other hand, Kanshin-Method made it possible to use much thinner needles to insert smoothly, as it uses Shinkan, a guide tube, to prevent needle bending, as the needle cannot bend more than the diameter of the tube. Kanshin-Method made Japanese practitioners start using extra thin, and smooth painless insertion for patients' comfort became standard in Japan. The insertion stimulation does not need to be such a painful process, as Japanese believe treatment efficacy is not depending on insertion pain, but rather by grasping and moving Ki. Further, constant improvement on Japanese needle manufacturing technology contributed to Japanese Shinkan technology, as it changed the standard of needle choice and insertion method dramatically in Shinkyu. Generally speaking, commonly used needles in Japan are so thin at 0.12-0.26mm diameters. In China, needles thinner than 0.30mm are rarely used clinically. Many practitioners, teachers and patients believe one of the major differences between the Japanese Shinkyu and Chinese style acupuncture is the needle thickness: Japanese tend to use extra thin needles, and Chinese use thicker ones. In Japan, the invention of Kanshin-Method using extra thin needles

Acupuncture Needle Gage Chart in Japan

Diameter	Japanese General Gage Numbers (Gou)	Japanese Gage Numbers (Ban*)	Chinese Gage Numbers (Gou)
0.12 MM	12 (Gou)	02(00) (Ban*)	
0.14 MM	14 (Gou)	01 (Ban*)	
0.16 MM	16 (Gou)	1 (Ban*)	
0.18 MM	18 (Gou)	2 (Ban*)	
0.20 MM	20 (Gou)	3 (Ban*)	
0.22 MM	22 (Gou)	4 (Ban*)	35 (Gou)
0.24 MM	24 (Gou)	5 (Ban*)	34 (Gou)
0.26 MM	26 (Gou)	6 (Ban*)	33 (Gou)
0.28 MM	28 (Gou)	7 (Ban*)	32 (Gou)
0.30 MM	30 (Gou)	8 (Ban*)	31 (Gou)
0.32 MM	32 (Gou)	9 (Ban*)	30 (Gou)
0.34 MM	34 (Gou)	10 (Ban*)	29 (Gou)
0.38 MM	38 (Gou)		28 (Gou)
0.42 MM	42 (Gou)		27 (Gou)
0.45 MM	45 (Gou)		26 (Gou)

*Commonly used for acupuncture

became a revolution in the history of acupuncture, and changed the daily clinical practice. It all started in the seventeenth century, so this time was the beginning of modern Japanese Shinkyu.

Currently, there are so many Shinkyu styles and schools available in Japan, and there is not one "standardized" method or technique to represent the whole Japanese Shinkyu. All styles and schools that are stemmed from any era in Japan can be called Japanese Shinkyu. But commonly, almost all Japanese styles, methods and schools use Kanshin-Method, with extra thin needles: thus, we can say usage of extra thin needles and using Shinkan, which means using Kanshin-Method is symbolic to Japanese acupuncture style. This needle insertion method is now becoming a world standard as Kanshin-Method has been spreading all over the world these days. Kanshin-Method and extra thin needle usage was created through the ardent passion and constant relentless efforts made by

Waichi Sugiyama, the eastern medicine master who devoted his life to healthy and safe development of acupuncture technology in the seventeen century. The Kanshin-Method, originally from Japan, is becoming the leading needling method in the world nowadays. Due to his legacy, Waichi Sugiyama is known worldwide as the "father of Japanese acupuncture."

In Japan, the needle gage system is standardized. One standardized gage counting method used for all needle types including sewing needles and others. The system is somewhat similar to those of Chinese ones, but cannot apply the same gage numbers as Chinese gage numbers as Japanese do not use the same thickness range. Japanese needle gage number (counted "Gou" in Japanese) starts at 10 (0.10mm thickness), and numbers are increasing in every 0.02mm, and ends at 50 (0.50mm thickness). In total 21 standard gage numbers exist between 10-50 in Japan. For example, 10-Gou gage diameter is 0.10mm, and 11-Gou gage is 0.12mm diameter, 12-Gou is 0.14mm, and so on.

Further, a second needle gage system exists in Japan to emphasis the diameter of the needles and is mainly used in medicine including acupuncture. In this system, the gage is counted as "Ban," and is similar to the "Gou" system above, the number is increased every 0.02mm. But in this "Ban" system, gage counts from 01 and numbers are increased from there. In Japan, commonly used Ban is 02-Ban (0.12mm) to 08-Ban (0.30mm) for acupuncture. This "Ban" system is used more often in clinical and educational settings. Further, Japanese disposable acupuncture needle handle colors are differentiated by gage for easy identification for practitioners.

Sensitive and Detailed

Japanese Shinkyu have always had a high reputation for its sensitive, detailed treatment. These are quite important aspects of practicing acupuncture and moxibustion in Japan: we practitioners insert needles to someone's body, which can be quite a fearful and invasive experience if we do not act with sensitivity, and using fire for moxibustion can be quite dangerous too. In each action, Japanese practitioner tends to be extremely

detailed and sensitive to the patient's response. There are more eastern medicine practitioners outside of Japan who would love to learn Japanese style for this reason. Whenever facial cosmetic acupuncture was taught overseas, so many attendees wanted to learn not only the cosmetic acupuncture techniques, but also to obtain more knowledge about the sensitivity of Japanese Shinkyu because sensitive, detailed treatment is not only safer and more effective, but also more comfortable for patients.

Trusted "Japanese Quality"

From his long and frequent overseas visits, the author Kitagawa learned that everywhere he went, when people heard "Japanese," "made in Japan," "from Japan," they immediately feel safe, secure and believe it is first-class quality. For example, home electronic items, automobile, watch are not products invented by Japanese, yet Japan-made products enjoy top level reputation in each field, and "made in Japan" became a world-class brand. As a country, it is quite exclusive to establish a status like this. When tourists visit Japan, they also tend to be impressed by detailed and perfect high-quality service such as transportation system, convenience stores, etc., as well. With this current situation, we believe Japan-made Shinkyu can be a synonym of Japanese first-class quality eastern medicine in the world.

Extremely Clean and Hygienic

It is often said by overseas visitors that Japan and the Japanese are "extremely clean everywhere." Many are impressed by the spotless cleanness of public toilets and bathrooms. From infection control point of view, spotless cleanness is absolutely necessary aspect for eastern medicine practitioners. In Japan, it is one of the most important check points for public health center inspections and occupational educations. One example of the Japanese obsession for cleanness is the usage of disposable acupuncture needles. In Shinkyu practice, as we insert needles directly into skin, preventing infectious diseases, especially blood-borne ones such as

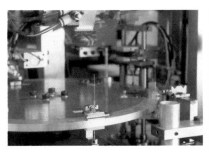
Manufacturing process of Japanese disposable acupuncture needles (Photo by Seirin)

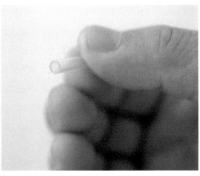
A Shinkan attached to a disposable acupuncture needle

HIV, HBV (Hepatitis B) and HCV (Hepatitis C) is an important aspect in clinical training and every day practice. In old times, acupuncture needles were used multiple times after being sterilized by autoclave. But due to the high awareness of infectious risks, Japan started using stainless single-use disposable needles ahead of most countries. Seirin, one of the most respected acupuncture medical manufacturers from Japan, was the first one to launch mass-produced single-use disposable acupuncture needles as early as 1978 in Japan. Since then, even though there is no Clean Needle Technique (which is a mandatory practice for licensed acupuncturists in the United States) educational requirement in Japan, it is rare to see any acupuncture clinics in Japan who does not use single-use stainless acupuncture needles in a perfectly clean, hygienic way. Also, Seirin, as the first company to offer stainless single-use disposable acupuncture needles to the world, has been exporting these needles to North America and Europe since the early days of disposable needles. These made-in-Japan clean single-use disposable needles changed the image of acupuncture practice to be much cleaner, safer, and thus helped the increase the demand in many countries. So we can say that Japanese Shinkyu, with our advanced manufacturing technology, contributed to the progress of acupuncture's clean clinical practice by offering tools for higher hygienic standard globally. Nowadays, stainless single-use disposable needles became a basic standard of acupuncture practice worldwide. Seirin has been the only

Japanese manufacturer who still manufactures all high-quality needles in Japan since early days, and its sophisticated technology made it possible to make their needle tips to be curved microscopically in order to avoid puncturing blood vessels and damage organs, as well as the insertion feeling to be rather smooth and more comfortable for patients. Most of its needles are coming with individual Shinkan, a guide tube, with handle which is color coded for easy recognition in the clinical environment. We will discuss more about Shinkan in the later chapters. Color-coding is particularly useful for practitioners who are in North America where the needle gage system is not easy to memorize. Many practitioners and students easily refer Seirin needles by handle colors ("I often use Seirin red ones," "we use Seirin light blue needles at school clinic," etc.). Such sophistications and detailed work come with high quality, advanced technologies and the Kanzen spirit how to be more hygienic and make cleaner environment. Japanese acupuncture clinics are often described as spotlessly clean and very hygienic including all tools, towels and they often offer well-cleaned gown/robe to wear for each treatment. Such detailed considerations represent the fine works of Japanese Shinkyu.

Sophisticated Skills and Manner

Historically, Japan is known for its unique adaptation skill: as a nation consisting of small islands, it has been adapting a lot of other culture, religions, language, knowledge and skills from neighbors and friends, and evolved them to be the "Japanese ways." Many of these imported technologies evolved and changed actually became more sophisticated and higher qualities - such as electronics, automobiles, trains, etc. This may suggest that Japanese may not be very good at bringing dynamic innovation from scratch, or the original thinkers, but they tend to be excelling at perfecting what they import and adapt. Shinkyu was also developed to became very Japanese with its long history, and nowadays it is often described as sophisticated eastern medicine as a combination of high technology, sensitive high-quality service with exquisite cleanness and detailed needling skills.

Globally, Japanese Shinkyu may not be known as most commonly practiced eastern medicine style, although it is becoming more known among licensed practitioners for its trusted quality, sensitive and detailed skill sets. As explained earlier in this chapter, Kanshin-Method using extra-thin needles, and single-use disposable needles all represent what make Japanese Shinkyu so unique and different. In the next chapters, we will explore the historical facts back in seventeenth century as this time was the pivotal moment for Japanese acupuncture development. This time was the birth place of the current modern Japanese Shinkyu. Waichi Sugiyama was the father of Japanese acupuncture, his life-long devotion to Japanese acupuncture development brought dynamic changes in acupuncture technology, technique, safety and knowledge.

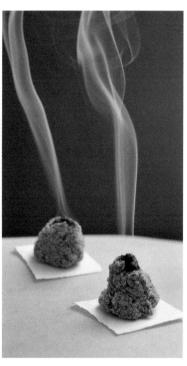

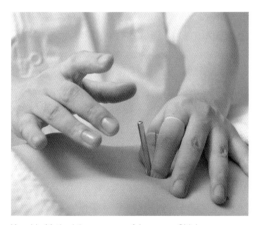

Kanshin Method the essence of Japanese Shinkyu

O-kyu; moxibustion is always integrated with acupuncture

Chapter 3

Acupuncture and Ki

Feel and Manipulate Ki

Waichi Sugiyama put the utmost priority to manage Ki in his acupuncture style. As you may be aware, Ki has always been the center of traditional east Asian medicine, Waichi repeatedly taught the importance for eastern medicine practitioners to acquire an ability to feel and manage Ki in the body. In his textbook "Sugiyama Shin Den Ryu (Sugiyama Style True Tradition)," he repeatedly stated "diagnosing Ki, and treating Ki are the objectives of acupuncture treatment."

There are considered to be two types of Ki : the first group is called vital energy (also simply just called Ki) which is also referred to as an energy force for all living creatures. There are several sub-types of different Ki flows in different meridians/areas of the body, such as "Grain Ki," "True Ki," "Protective Ki," etc. They are all the positive energy forces which maintain life. The second Ki group called "Jaki" in Japanese (Ja means evil or obstructive). Jaki group is known as "pathogenic factors" or "Evil Ki" in English, it is a group of negative energy which obstructs and interrupts the life force energy. There are six types of Jaki, Wind, Cold, Heat, Dampness, Dryness and Summer Heat – they are all invasive and affect our body negatively. Most of the time, they invade the body from the outside environment, such as climates, temperature, etc., but some may occur from internal causes, such as emotions, food and stress, etc. When we say Ki, it normally indicates the first group of vital energy Ki.

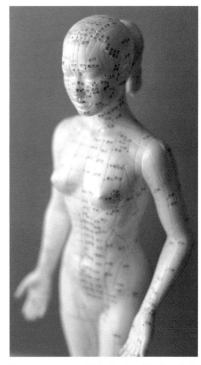

Meridian system – Ki is circulated in the whole body

Ki is circulating in our body thoroughly through the channels called meridians, which is called "Keiraku" in Japanese. Meridian is the original concept coming from eastern traditional medicine to address the paths of Ki, which has never existed in western medicine. Unlike modern medicine which is based on observable facts, both Ki and meridians cannot be seen nor examined by naked eyes. The word meridian consists of two Chinese characters 経絡. The first character 経 means wide vertical main roads or highways, and the second character 絡 represents narrower horizonal streets. These meridian characters can be referred to as the perfect representation of Ki's traffic system. Using the wide main highways and narrow streets, Ki can go anywhere freely throughout the body. Ki is circulating throughout our body by this meridian transportation system. Blood is following everywhere Ki goes to nourish our body.

In eastern medicine, healthy state is considered to be able to remove any pathogenic factors (Jaki) naturally, and once the obstruction is gone, the body recovers free Ki circulation. For example, when a town is invaded by outsiders, first to eliminate the enemy from the town, then to supply foods and necessary materials to regain the peace. In our body, the system recognizes Jaki, pathogenic factors as enemies, and the food supply is Ki and Blood.

In Japan, the official medicine was almost entirely replaced by modern western medicine in the time of Meiji restoration, the current medicine is not concerned about the existence of Ki or Jaki. However, the word Ki is still widely used in everyday language in Japan. As the word Ki is considered as a main noun to express emotion, feeling and energy, it is used more often in health. For example, feeling sick in Japanese is "Kimochi ga warui" (Ki is held poorly), and being unconscious is "Ki wo ushinau" (losing Ki) or "Kizetsu" (ki is out), and feeling well or full of energy is "genki" (ki is as good as it is originally)

Following the modern western medicine standard in Japan, recent acupuncture educational and clinical environment tend to emphasize anatomical and physiological knowledge over the importance of Ki. However, for thousands of years, acupuncture has been a major part of medicine, and managing Ki is a fundamental practice. Throughout the centuries,

including ancient China and seventeen century Japan when Waichi Sugiyama treated thousands of patients, the eastern medical system healed millions of people without advanced detailed knowledge of pathophysiology, blood test or X-ray, which is what the modern western medical system has developed into. However, in the eastern medical system, it is absolutely essential to sense, diagnose and manage the Ki energy of each patient. Many modern Japanese medical practitioners look like they have forgotten about this, but it is important for us, eastern medical practitioners to be aware that modern western medical knowledge is important, but not everything. By learning Sugiyama Style Acupuncture Jutsu, an art of knowledge and technique, you can recognize (or re-recognize) the fundamental philosophy of "sense, grasp and move Ki is the goal of acupuncture treatment" – very basic, but tends to be forgotten in the modern era of technology and science. Through this book, you will never forget the importance of recognizing and managing Ki.

Acupuncture's Efficacy for Ki

In the book Sugiyama Shin Den Ryu, which is the center of the School of Sugiyama Style, he reveals the five important actions of acupuncture treatment: 1) to give Hibiki sensation, 2) to tonify, 3) to drain/disperse and 4) move/induce Ki, and last but not least, 5) harmonize the body. Especially, Waichi Sugiyama made a special emphasis that acupuncture's goal should be bringing the "Ki arrival" on the needling site via the Hibiki sensation. First, let's talk through what Hibiki is.

1). Hibiki – the Arrival of Ki

Acupuncture needle stimulation sensation is very unique and specific to acupuncture treatment. It can often be described by patients as dull, heavy, sore and/or numbing/tingling feeling. This special feeling is called "De-Qi" in China, which means the arrival of Ki. The Chinese word is directly used as-is in English, as western medicine does not have a direct translation. This unique acupuncture sensation is called Hibiki in Japanese.

Hibiki literally means a sound, vibration or ring in Japanese. In acupuncture, it means the arrival of Ki, and can be similar feeling as De-Qi, or can be somewhat milder and gentler, as Japanese tend to use thinner needles and needling depth can often be shallower. This special feeling is coming from physiological responses via needle insertion or manipulation on site. As stated in the earlier chapter, in Chinese acupuncture, much thicker and longer needles are used than in Japan, plus the needling method is rather direct, as Nen-Shin method (where the needle is inserted without using the guide tube,) is used, this sensation could be quite strong. In Japanese acupuncture style, in general the needle insertion tends to be gentler by using thinner needles with Shinkan, so Hibiki can be softer or lighter. This type of sensation may be varied, as it is a unique response by individuals, plus also depending on the day, health condition and/or needling method, etc. So, you can see that Hibiki is generally considered as a unique sensation created by Japanese style acupuncture – using thinner needles, Shinkan and shallow insertion.

As stated earlier, modern medicine does not concern itself much about the existence of Ki, so even in the Japanese traditional medicine field, the understanding and recognition of Ki and Hibiki have been somewhat diluted in the clinical and educational environment. However, the arrival of Ki is considered one of the most important responses directly connected to treatment efficacy since ancient time in China. As Waichi Sugiyama learned the classic acupuncture medicine rooted in ancient time, in the Sugiyama Style acupuncture, Hibiki is an important element of every treatment. Waichi repeatedly said "when giving acupuncture treatment, recognize the Ki and make sure of the Ki arrival. This is the one and only indicator of efficacious treatment." This statement indicates that when you cannot let Ki arrive, there is no efficacy in that treatment unfortunately. The arrival of Ki which is felt as the feeling of Hibiki, is the direct physiological response coming from acupuncture needling, and the most important factor of acupuncture treatment efficacy.

The term "arrival of Ki" has two indications: one is to circulate Ki to the diseased area locally, and for the patient to feel Hibiki on the needling site as the "arrival" of Ki. For example, when there is pain due to the local

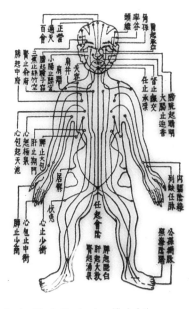

Ancient illustration to show Ki cirulation

obstruction by evil Ki or pathogenic factors, needling can bring Ki to arrive on site to remove the pathogens, and as a consequence, alleviate pain. So, the arrival of Ki can be local. Another indication of Ki arrival is that the patient feels the whole body getting re-energized and feeling refreshed after treatment. In the classic Chinese literature Ling Shu Chapter 1 (nine needles and 12 sources) states that the essential point for needling is that when the Qi (Ki) arrives and treatment is effective, it feels as "wind blows away the clouds and it is clear like seeing the blue sky".

Further, Waichi Sugiyama's book states that evil Ki arrives fast, and on arrival, acupuncture needle feel tension and can sense a tingling feeling underneath the needled area. On the other hand, Ki arrives slowly and feels soft and warm on arrival on the site. This statement indicates it may take more than a few seconds for Ki to arrive underneath the needling point. Then from there, Ki circulates and spreads to the whole body. We can say that Hibiki is the first response of the body for feeling Ki arrival locally, then it slowly spreads to the entire body from there. As Ki arrives with Hibiki, if there is no Hibiki, there would be no Ki arrival on site, so most likely it would not spread to the whole body, meaning no efficacy of the treatment. It is important to ensure each patient, with Hibiki, feels the arrival of Ki with a warm, soft feeling on the needling site and later feels the whole body to be recharged or refreshed after the treatment (although it may take time to feel it). For your note, as the arrival of Ki may take time, acupuncturists almost always retain needles on patients during acupuncture treatment. This is to make sure the Ki arrival occurs during every treatment.

2). Tonifying – Circulating Ki and Blood

A town can be slowly deserted or ruined when there is no traffic, no residents and people around. The human body can also be negatively affected by deficiency of Ki circulation. Ki should be freely circulated in the entire body throughout the body's network system called meridians. The area where Ki is deficient can also be deficient in Blood, due to that Blood following where Ki flows. Acupuncture can restore and promote Ki circulation or fill up the Ki where it is deficient. When Ki flows, Blood follows, so acupuncture to treat Ki is also promoting Blood to circulate and deliver nourishment to the body.

3). Draining Ki - Dispel Evil Ki

On the contrary to deficiency, a town with constant heavy traffic jams and too many people is not considered healthy, as such fullness creates more accidents and stagnation in streets, and may increase pollution and crime and create an unhealthy environment. When our body has too much fullness or obstruction, Ki gets stagnated and cannot circulate freely. This is called Ki Stagnation, and acts as an unhealthy by-product bringing negative outcomes such as pain, taut band, muscle knots or diseases – often causing local inflammations. Acupuncture can disperse or dispel such Ki Stagnation so the body regains the healthy traffic of Ki. Alternatively, pathogens from outside (such as Wind, Cold, Dryness, etc.) can enter the body and start obstructing the flow of Ki. Acupuncture can dispel and drain such outside evils and recover the Ki and Blood circulation in the body.

4). Induction: Move Ki to the Meridian Ends and/or Inside/out Parts of the Body

When body has evil Ki: pathogenic factors within the body's core can cause pain, acupuncture can move such evil pathogens to the extremities by needling the tips of the hands or feet (that are normally the end of meridian networks). Also, when the abdomen or any front part of the body is diseased, acupuncture can guide such pathogenic factors to move to the

back area of the body by needling the back, and eventually dispel the pathogens, then abdominal signs and symptoms can be improved or disappeared. Acupuncture can aim to dispel evil pathogens out of the diseased area by needling opposite or other parts of the body. Such acupuncture needling jutsu to guide/induce Ki to move from one area to another is called "Hikibari" in Japanese (pulling Ki from one area to another).

5). Harmony of Ki and Blood

One of acupuncture's great benefits is to harmonize the body. This means to balance the body's homeostasis. For eastern medicine practitioners, harmonized body means that body has a good Yin-Yang balance. As we all learned at school, Ki is Yang, Blood is Yin, and thus Yin-Yang balance means Ki and Blood are well harmonized. This harmony can be achieved by Hibiki, by using a combination of Tonifying, Draining and Induction which we addressed in this chapter. Depending on the presentation of the patient, you may use one of them or all combined, to bring a harmony to the patient's body. When patients fall asleep during treatment and/or feels refreshed, that's the manifestation of the arrival of Ki and harmony. As stated earlier in this chapter, Lin Shu describes perfectly what the harmony feels like "as if wind blows aways the clouds" and it is to see the blue sky.

As mentioned, the goal of acupuncture is to manage Ki. This can be done by sending, detecting, regulating and moving Ki and pathogenic factors. Practitioners must purposefully aim to make "Hibiki" plus use appropriate jutsu such as "tonify," "drain" and/or "induce" Ki to bring the result: the patient must feel the arrival of Ki, and after treatment, feel energized or refreshed as improved healthy, better Ki and Blood circulation and the whole body is harmonized. As both Ki and pathogens cannot be seen by the naked eye, it is necessary for practitioners to acquire "sensing" and "detecting" Ki flow in meridians. The Sugiyama Style emphasizes this fundamental concept and repeated the importance of "diagnose and manage Ki." We believe it is a mandatory to learn and understand the Sugiyama Style Acupuncture.

Chapter 4

Kanshin Needling Method

To the World Standard Needling Method

As we addressed at the beginning of this book, Kanshin Method is not considered as a needling skill, but rather as "the total acupuncture methodology Jutsu using Shinkan (guide tube)," including needling techniques utilizing Shinkan. Hence, in this chapter, we talk about two sections: one is Kanshin Needling Method focusing on needling skill, and another one is Kanshin Jutsu which is about more broad practice including non-needling techniques utilizing Shinkan.

Kanshin Needling Method

As stated, Kanshin Method is one of the needling methods to use a Shikan (guide tube) to insert every needle. When people use the phrase Kanshin Method, it usually indicates this specific needling method in Japan. This has been the standard needling method in Japanese clinical and educational environments for a long time. Nowadays, Kanshin needling method has become a world standard as many non-Japanese acupuncturists use guide tubes as a default needling method.

●Shinkan (guide tube)

In Japan, the mainstream method is to use stainless disposable acupuncture needles. In each disposable needle pack, a plastic guide tube (Shinkan) comes with it. Shinkan used to be made of stainless steel or silver, but nowadays is made of plastic and can be disposable too.

Needling Hand ("Sashi-de") and Supporting Pushing Hand ("Oshi-de")

In traditional Chinese needling method, called as Nen-Shin-Method in Japanese, as we discussed in the previous chapter, the whole needling

Kanshin Method Needle Setting – "Sou-Kan" ("inserting in a tube")

process is done by one hand. In Kanshin needling method, needling is usually done by using both hands: one hand to hold or "push" the skin of the needling site firmly, while the other hand inserts the needle. In Kanshin needling method, this "pushing" hand is called "Oshi-de"(Oshi comes from the verb means "push" in Japanese) and the needling hand is called "Sashi-de" (Sashi comes from a verb meaning "needling") in Japanese.

In his book "Sugiyama Shin Den Ryu (Sugiyama Style True Tradition)," fourteen types of Oshi-de were introduced. However, there are some types that are not really applicable for modern time practice any more, hence we do not explain each of them: "Full moon" and "Half-moon" Oshi-de types are used most commonly in this book.

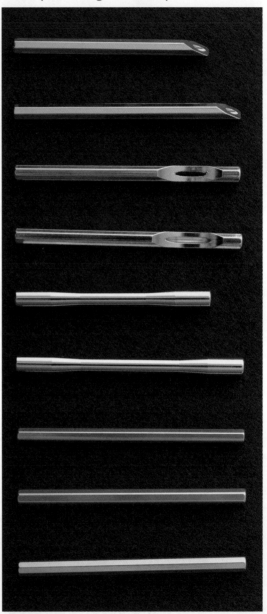

Various types of Shinkan (full size)

Full Moon Oshi-de (pushing hand)

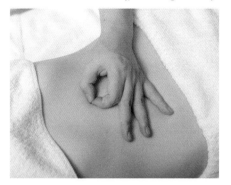

Make a circle (full moon) by the thumb and index finger and press the palm. The rest of the fingers are straight and pressed against the skin. This is commonly used when needling perpendicularly.

Half Moon Oshi-de (pushing hand)

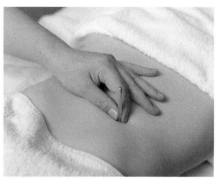

Make a half-circle by the straight thumb and curled index fingers. The rest of the fingers are kept straight. This is commonly used when needling transversely or obliquely.

Needling Setting to Shinkan

The process where a needle is set to the Shinkan is called "Sou-Kan" ("inserting to a tube"). There are two types of insertion styles; two-hands setting and one-hand setting. However, these days many commercial acupuncture needles are packaged as pre-set in Shinkan (the individual needles are already set into the guide tubes), so these setting skills are becoming less focused in the process of modern time acupuncture. However, some acupuncture needles are pre-packaged as one Shinkan per 5-10 needles or more, so efficiently and safely inserting needle into Shinkan each time is still a skill for effective treatment.

◎ Two-hands Setting Method

The needling hand holds the Shinkan, then the pushing hand inserts the needle into the Shinkan: once set, hold the Shinkan and the needle inside together firmly, not letting the tip of the needle stick out of the Shinkan.

◎ One-hand Setting Method

One-hand Soukan setting is done only by using the needling hand, and

Two-hands Insertion

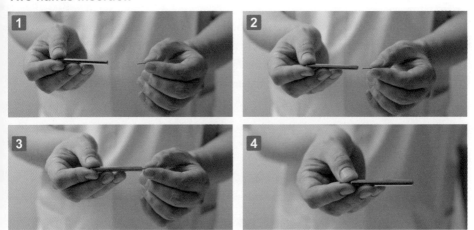

1. One hand holds the needle handle, the other hand holds an empty Shinkan – both horizontally.
2. The handle of the needle to be horizontally inserted into the Shinkan.
3. Adjust the Shinkan angle to make the needle handle just come out the other end of the Shinkan, approximately around 2-3mm.   This protrusion is called "Dragon's Head."
4. Pinch the protruding needle handle with the thumb and index finger, and hold the Shinkan by the remaining fingers.

One-hand Insertion

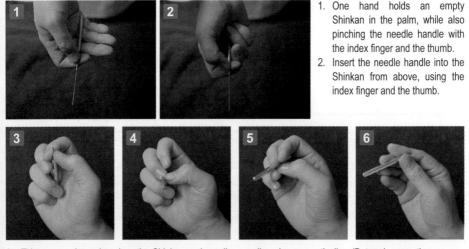

1. One hand holds an empty Shinkan in the palm, while also pinching the needle handle with the index finger and the thumb.
2. Insert the needle handle into the Shinkan from above, using the index finger and the thumb.

3. This process is easier when the Shinkan and needle are aligned more vertically. (But make sure the needle does not fall out the other end.)
4. Place Shinkan on the middle finger joint
5. Turn the Shinkan (needle is in it) at 90-degree on the middle finger (vertical to horizontal)
6. Pinch the tip of the needle handle to ready to needle.

this is the most commonly used method to set the needle inside the Shinkan. It requires practice and is relatively challenging for the beginners, but it is a very fast and efficient method. In Japanese acupuncture schools, this one-hand setting method is a must-have skill for all acupuncture students.

Seppi (Needle incision) and Dan-nyu (Needle Incision Procedure)

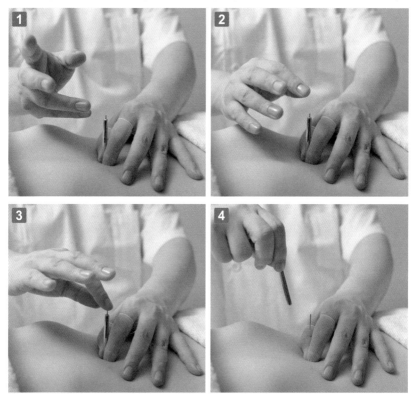

1. Place the Shinkan, with the needle set inside, vertically on the skin. (the handle of the needle is protruded 2-3mm above the Shinkan – which is also called the "Dragon's Head.")
2nd & 3rd pictures: tap gently 3 – 5 times on the head of the needle to insert into the skin.
4. Sashi-de (needling hand) to remove the needle, while Oshi-de (pushing hand) holds the needle lightly.

Seppi (incision) and Dan-nyu (incision technique)

With its long history of acupuncture practice and keenness on following precise procedure and techniques, there are several Japanese keywords to describe the process of the needle being inserted into the skin. One is Seppi which means incision, a moment when a needle is inserted in the skin, and another is Dan-nyu which is a technique to make the insertion into the skin.

◎ Dan-nyu

On the site where you want to insert the needle, hold the Shikan by the thumb and index finger of the pushing hand. Then the index finder of the needling hand taps gently to insert the needle into the skin.

◎ Needle Insertion

After Dan-nyu (tapping in the needle), Seppi is done. Then, there are two ways to move the needle into the skin a little deeper, this is commonly practiced in Japan: Sending Method and Sen-Nen Method.

Sending Method

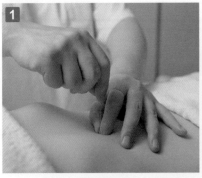 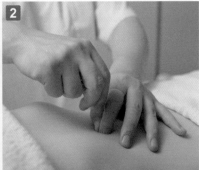

1. The needle is inserted. Oshi-de (pushing hand) supports the site (and needle) for stability.
2. The needle is gradually inserted deeper by Sashi-de (needling hand).

●Sending Method

Holding a needle by the thumb and the index finger of the needling hand, then apply a force to "send" the needle underneath the skin.

●Sen-Nen Method

Holding a needle by the thumb and the index finder of the needling hand, then apply a force to push the needle in, while rotating the needle tip right or left between 120 to 180 degrees.

Sen-Nen Method

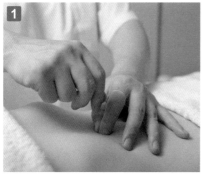 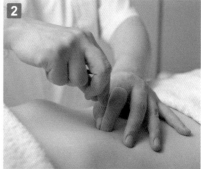

1. Holding a needle by the thumb and the index finder of the Sashi-de (needling hand), then push the needle in, while rotating to the right.
2. Rotating the needle to the left. Continue to rotate right to left, left to right while deepening the needle.

Chapter 5

The Fourteen

Kan Jutsu

Purpose and Classification of The Fourteen Kan Jutsu

The fourteen Kan Jutsu were created by Waichi Sugiyama in the seventeenth century. The invention of the Shinkan (guide tube) elevated acupuncture to the next level. These Kan jutsu give additional stimulations to the needling site, by using the Shinkan as a tool. There are fourteen types of different jutsu, with different objectives and techniques, and each gives significant benefit to patients.

The overall major objectives and effect of The Fourteen Kan Jutsu are to strengthen the benefits of acupuncture needling to manage Ki, such as Hibiki (Ki arrival), Tonifying, Draining (or some may say Reducing or Dispersing), Moving/Inducing and Harmonizing, as we learned in the previous chapters. Also, The Fourteen Kan Jutsu spreads needling effects to the surrounding area of the needling site to enhance treatment efficacy.

◎ Summary of the objectives:

①.Strengthening the needling effects – Tonifying, Draining, Moving/Inducing and Harmonizing
②.Spreading the Hibiki and stimulations on the needling site and surrounding areas

The Fourteen Kan Jutsu can broadly be divided into four groups. In this chapter, the characteristics, effects and clinical applications of each jutsu are explained. Further, each technique and specific clinical example are discussed so readers can practice them from today. Further, when each of these fourteen jutsu are analyzed in detail, there are similarities in some of the techniques and objectives: we address these commonalities and differences in this chapter as well, so each jutsu can be clearly distinguished and applied in a clinical setting.

Also, as explained in Chapter3, there are some objectives of

acupuncture needling, such as to give Hibiki, which is an arrival of Ki in Japanese, plus, give needling efficacies such as tonify, drain/disperse, move/induce Ki and/or giving harmony to the entire body. Some of the jutsu can give extensive effects such as strengthening, propagation, etc. They are addressed in this chapter. Further, each clinical application addresses the strategic acupuncture points to use, so readers can clearly understand how to use each jutsu and the reason for each usage.

Note: for clarity, in this book, each jutsu is explained using the perpendicular needling method.

◎ The Fourteen Kan Jutsu Groups

①.Tapping Kan Jutsu
  Fine Finger Kan, Rising Sun Kan, Ki Tapping Kan

②.Needle Pressing Kan Jutsu
  Finger Pressing Kan, Tube Pressing Kan

③.Surround Tapping and Scrubbing Kan Jutsu
  Tapping Around Kan, Spring Finger Kan, Far Sense Kan, Muscle Rubbing Kan

④.Needle Vibration Kan Jutsu
  Dragon's Head Kan, Ingenious Dragon's Head Kan, Glowing Needle Kan, Internal Tuning Kan, Connecting Valley Kan

1. Tapping Kan Jutsu

Fine Finger Kan, Rising Sun Kan, Ki-tapping Kan

【 Main Effects 】
The tapping techniques can seem similar in their concepts among the

three Kan jutsu; however, each objective and benefit is clearly different as below:

Fine Finger Kan : drain and disperse the Evil Heat on the surface of the skin

Rising Sun Kan : pull the Evil Heat residing deep inside the body (and drain it)

Ki Tapping Kan : spread the Hibiki around the needling site more widely

【 Similarities and Differentiations 】

The common technique between Fine Finger Kan jutsu and Rising Sun Kan jutsu is tapping on the top of the Shinkan. But while Fine Finger Kan taps just the needle head protruding above the Shinkan or tip of the Shinkan, Rising Sun Kan taps the whole Shinkan when the needle is already inserted in the body. Plus, Ki Tapping Kan is unique by itself: it taps the head of the Shinkan when it is placed by the side of the inserted needle.

◎ Fine Finger Kan

●The origin of the name

It was named as the finger to tap the head of the needle protruded from the Shinkan many times at very fine, fast rhythm.

●Main effect

Disperse the Evil Ki stagnated underneath the skin surface (draining method).

●How to hold the Shinkan

Hold the tip of Shinkan at the bottom by the thumb and the index finger of the Oshi-de (pushing hand).

●Technique

Place the needle at the target site, and give gentle, fast taps to the

Fine Finger Kan

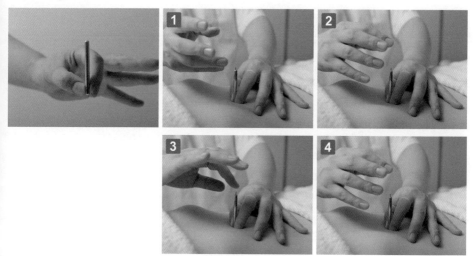

1. Place the needle at the target site.
2. Give very light, gentle taps at very fast, fine rhythm for 100-200 times at the Dragon's Head – the protruded head of the needle from the Shinkan.
3. Keep tapping. If the needle is inserted, it is ok, just tap the head of Shinkan.
4. If you can tap faster and give more taps, it is better as more stimulation is given to the site.

protruded head of the needle from the Shinkan (this head is also called "Dragon Head"). The needle can be inserted by the first 3-5 taps, but keep tapping the head of Shinkan with a very fast, fine rhythm for 100-200 times. If you can tap faster and give more taps, it is better as it gives more stimulation to the site. In this jutsu. It is not about deepening the needle insertion depth by giving more taps, It is important to give light taps to the head of Shinkan after the needle is inserted.

•Clinical Usage Examples:
- Use for cold or influenza fever, chill, stiff or painful neck, shoulder and/or back (draining method). Acupuncture points can be varied depending on the condition.
- Use for the whole Trapezius muscle to release surface muscle tensions, stiffness, etc., and promote sweating to disperse Cold/Wind Evils (draining method).
- When there is a tearing and/or red, itchy eyes, use this method for BL2

(Zanzhu) (draining method).

- When there is an amenorrhea related to Blood Stagnation/depression, use for KD6 (Zhaohai) or BL67 (Zhiyin) (induction).
- For postpartum chest and/or abdominal pain, use for PC6 (Neiguan) (induction).

◎ Rising Sun Kan

●The origin of the name

Named as the rising sun, this jutsu gives the effect gradually, as if the sun is gradually rising in the morning. It is to tap the Shinkan in a step-by-step manner, and disperse the Evil Heat residing deep in the body.

Rising Sun Kan

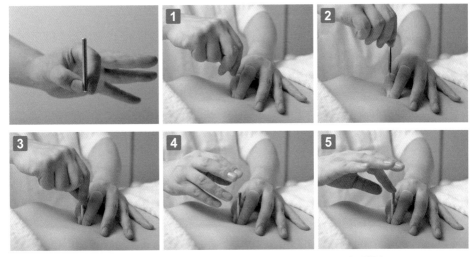

1. Place the needle at the target site and insert to around 4-5mm depth, and remove the Shinkan.
2. Make sure the needle is stable. Then put the Shinkan back over the needle.
3. Press the Shinkan on the skin.
4. Use the tip of index finger of Sashi-de (needling hand).
5. Tap the head of Shinkan with a fast, fine rhythm. Please make sure the tapping is enough at 30-50 times.

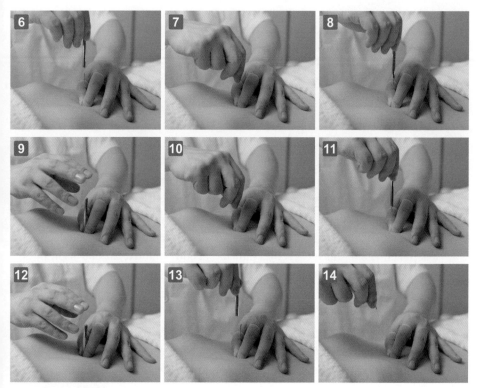

6. Remove the Shinkan.
7. Deepen the needle another 4-5mm.
8. Put the Shinkan back.
9. Tap again (see #5). Repeat the same process until the needle reaches the desired depth.
10. When it is done, pull the needle slightly, around 4mm.
11. Put the Shinkan back.
12. Tap the same way as #5 or #9.
13. Pull the needle 4-5mm each time until the needle depth is 2mm. Then remove the Shinkan.
14. Remove the needle.

•**Main effects**

Pull and raise the Evil Ki (Heat) to the surface and disperse it (draining method).

Promote Hibiki and circulate Ki and Blood (tonifying method) for chronic pain caused by either deficient or excess conditions.

●How to hold the Shinkan

Hold the Shinkan by thumb and index finger (same way as the Fine Finger Kan).

●Technique

Tap to insert the needle on the site, remove the Shinkan and make sure the needle insertion depth reaches around 4-5mm (so it is stable). Then put back the Shinkan over the needle and tap the Shinkan head at a fast, fine rhythm like Fine Finger Kan. Remove the Shinkan again and insert the needle a little deeper, put the Shinkan back and repeat the tapping. Repeat 2-3 times, each time going deeper until the needle reaches the desired depth.

When removing the needle, pull the needle slightly, around 4-5mm, and put back the Shinkan and tap the Shinkan head in fine rhythm, remove the Shinkan: repeat, pulling the needle 4-5mm each time until the needle depth is shallow at 2-3mm. Then do one last tap with Shinkan and remove the needle.

Note: Rising Sun Kan Jutsu is similar to what we call "Ji-Shi Needling method" which is taught widely in Japan today.

●Clinical Usage Examples:

- Disperse the Evil Heat from joint inflammation causing pains in the extremities (draining method). Desirable acupuncture points depend on the condition.
- Apply for abdomen or lower back points for amenorrhea, painful menstruation and/or low appetite (tonifying method).
- For pain or Evil Ki in the chest wall, induce them to the Jing-Well points through the relevant meridians (induction).
- Apply for SP9 (Yinlingquan) for leg and foot numbness (tonifying method).
- For pain in the medial side of foot or sole of the foot, first reat SP4 (Gongsun) and KD1(Yongquan), then apply for ST36 (ZuSanli) to improve the blood flow (tonifying method).
- Apply for CV4 (Guanyuan) for deficient conditions with Cold diseases (tonifying method).

- Apply for CV13 (Shangwan) for continuous hiccup (tonifying method).
- Apply for ST25 (Tianshu) for deficient diarrhea (tonifying method).
- Apply for SP6 (Sanyinjiao) to move down the abdomen Evil Ki causing postpartum abdominal pain and/or Blood Stagnation, after regulating Ki in abdomen (induction).

◎ Ki tapping Kan

●the origin of the name

The name comes from the technique to make the Ki arrive by fine tapping the Shinkan right next to the needle.

●Main Effects

After encouraging Hibiki, Ki-arrival, let the depressed Ki disperse so
the Ki is spread to the surrounding area (propagation).

Release the tensions of the large muscles (strengthening).

●How to Hold Shinkan

The tip of the Shinkan is held by the thumb and index fingers.

●Technique

Insert the needle into the targeted site at the targeted depth. Remove the
Shinkan. Place the shinkan right next to the inserted needle. Then the needle and Shinkan together are to be held by the thumb and the index finger
of Oshi-de (pushing hand). Then using the Sashi-de (needling hand) index
finger, tap the head of the Shinkan. Tap with fine, fast rhythm like Fine-
Finger Kan and Raising sun Kan jutsu.

After 3-4 breaths of fast tapping, move the Shinkan to a different angle
and tap in fine rhythm. After another 3-4 breaths, repeat and tap from
another angle. Repeat till finish tapping at all angles. After finishing all
tapping, immediately remove the needle.

The objective of this is to spread the Ki to the area surrounding the
needling site.

Ki tapping Kan

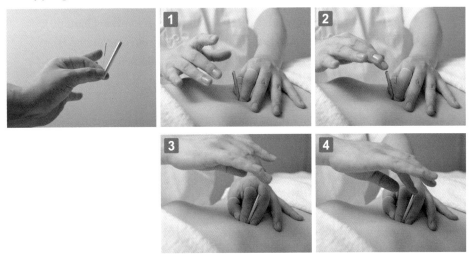

1. Insert the needle at the targeted depth. Remove the Shinkan. Place the Shikan right next to the inserted needle and hold together by the index finger and thumb of Oshi-de (pushing hand).
2. Then use Sashi-de (needling hand) to tap the head of Shinkan. Tap with fine, fast rhythm.
3. Pinch the Shinkan between the thumb and the middle finger (different angle).
4. Tap the head of Shinkan like #2. After giving enough tapping at different angles. Remove the needle and Shinkan.

●Clinical Usage Examples:

- Upper abdominal pain, side head pain, cold extremities, constricted muscles, muscle pain and/or cramping caused by the inflammation and cold.
- Apply for back Shu points, wide muscles such as temporalis muscle (TH20, Jiaosun), sole of the foot (KD1, Yongquan), and/or side of the leg (GB31, Fengshi) at the Tensor Fasciae latae.
o Back Shu points to regulate deficient Zang-Fu functions.
o TH20 (Jiaosun) for toothache (draining method).
o KD1 (Yongquan) for leg pain (draining method).
o GB31 (Fengshu) for leg and knee pain and cramps (strengthening).
o BL17 (Geshu) and BL18 (Ganshu) for regulating Liver functions, especially for postpartum bleeding (strengthening).

2. Needle Pressing Kan Jutsu

Finger Pressing Kan, Tube Pressing Kan

【 Main Effects 】
Spread the Ki and Blood to ease the tensions and constrictions in the deep area where the needle tip cannot reach

【 Clinical Applications 】
This jutsu is ideal for patients who are sensitive to needles and thus cannot be needled deeply, or for relatively young patients who receive acupuncture for the first time. Needling can be shallow, but with additional Shinkan stimulation, it releases the tensions or constrictions of the muscles deeper inside where the needle tip cannot reach.

【 Similarities and differences 】
Finger Pressing Kan and Tube Pressing Kan are similar jutsu: the only difference is whether to push the Shinkan with the needle set inside, or push it without.

◎ Finger Pressing Kan

●the Origin of the Name
This jutsu is to use fingers to press Shinkan and needle, hence called as Finger Pressing Kan.

●Main Effects
Dispersing Evil Ki (draining method).
Spreading K i and Blood (tonifying method).

●How to Hold a Shinkan
Using Oshi-de (pushing hand), hold the needle by the thumb and the

Finger Pressing Kan

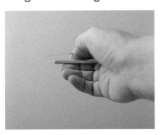

1. Insert the needle at the target depth. Remove Shinkan.
2. Place the Shinkan by Sashi-de (needling hand) right next to the needle and press the Shinkan on the skin.
3. Hold the needle handle by the thumb and the index finger of Sashi-de (needling hand), and use the middle finger joint to support the head of Shinkan.
4. Press both needle and Shinkan together by using both hands.
5. Repeated press and gently release, then press again, release.
6. When pressed enough times, remove the needle and Shinkan.

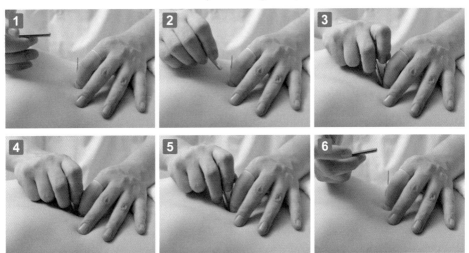

index finger and put Shinkan head between the middle finger's joint.

●Technique

Insert the needle shallower than the target depth. Remove Shinkan. Then hold the needle handle by the thumb and the index finger of Oshi-de (pushing hand). Place the Shinkan by Sashi-de (needling hand) right next to the needle, and hold the end of the Shinkan at the middle finger joint. Then press both the needle and Shinkan together by using both hands. Repeat the press and gently release, then press again, release. When pressed enough times and feel the Ki is spread, remove the needle and Shinkan.

●Clinical Usage Examples:

- When abdomen is cold and/or shows signs of Wind-Cold, apply for CV12 (Zhongwan) (tonifying method).
- For pain in lower abdomen and/or lower back, or heat/warm sensation by UTI inflammation, blood in urine or any local pain by Ki stagnations, apply for lower abdomen or lower back points (draining method). Strategic points are different depending on the presentation.
- Any abdominal pain below umbilicus, apply for SP6 (Sanyinjiao) and SP9 (Yinlingquan) (induction).
- For painful or cramping elbows, apply for LI9 (Shanglian) (tonifying method).

◎ Tube Pressing Kan

●the Origin of the Name

Named as Tube Pressing Kan as this method is to press and push the skin by Shinkan with needle set in. This is to give vertical pressing to enable Ki to be released from the deeper layers of the body.

●Main Effects

Release the muscular tensions a ort with the remaining fingers.

●How to Hold a Shinkan

Hold the end of the Shinkan by the thumb and the index finger of the Oshi-de (pushing hand) and support with the remaining fingers.

●Technique

Insert the needle to a desirable depth, then, keep the Shinkan over the needle. Press the Shinkan against the skin by using the index finger and thumb. Repeat as many times as you wish until you feel Ki release. Remove the Shinkan, manipulate the needle using a technique such as sparrow-pecking, etc., then place the Shinkan back and press again for further changes. Press as many times as you wish. Then remove the Shinkan and the needle.

Tube Pressing Kan

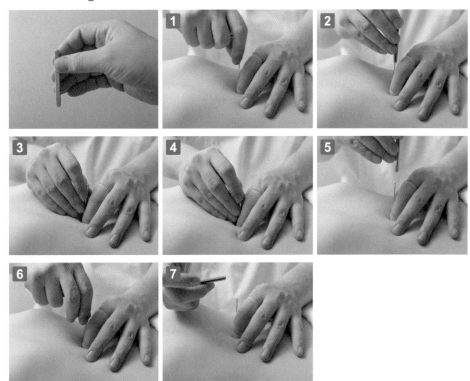

1. Insert the needle at desirable depth.
2. Place the Shinkan over the needle. (if needling is done with Shinkan, just keep it there.)
3. Make sure to press Shikan against the skin
4. Use both hands and press/push the Shinkan against the skin.
5. Remove the Shinkan only (leave the needle inserted)
6. Manipulate the needle using a technique such as sparrow-pecking, etc., and place the Shinkan back and press again (process #2-4)
7. When pressed enough times, remove the needle and Shinkan.

•Clinical Usage Examples: for both, specific acupuncture points are depending on the condition.

- Apply for relatively young patients to release the muscular tensions and constrictions with dried and fatigued eyes.
- Apply for relatively sensitive patients to release the deep muscular tensions and constrictions with abdominal and/or back pain for those who are sensitive to needling.

58

3. Surround Tapping and Scrubbing Kan Jutsu

Tapping Around Kan, Spring Finger Kan, Far Sense Kan and Muscle Rubbing Kan

【 Main Effects 】
① Alleviate pain and release muscular tensions by dispersing the Evil Ki (draining method)
② Release the muscular tensions by gathering and moving Ki and Blood around the needling site (tonifying method).

【 Clinical Application 】
- In general, use these jutsu for the pain coming from widely spread Ki stagnation and/or Evil Ki residence.
- Use Tapping Around Kan, Spring Finger Kan and Far-Sense Kan for painful areas with excess conditions with Evil Ki residence. These can also be used for deficient condition with cold constrictions. For the cold conditions, tap the Shinkan slowly with pushing motion to warm and release the muscles to circulate Ki and Blood.
- Further, Far-Sense Kan can enhance the draining method, and Muscle Rubbing Kan is used to enhance the tonifying method.

【 Jutsu Classifications 】
① Tapping around the needled site: Tapping Around Kan Jutsu, Spring Finger Kan Jutsu, and Far Sense Kan Jutsu
② Rubbing around the needled site: Muscle Rubbing Kan Jutsu

【 Similarities and differences 】
●**Tapping Around Kan and Spring Finger Kan**
These jutsu look similar in their objectives and the fact both of them tap around the needed site while the needle is inserted. However, Tapping Around Kan uses one Shinkan, and one hand, while Spring Finger Kan

uses two Shinkan (two guide tubes) together using both hands, like drumming a taiko.

●Spring Finger Kan and Far Sense Kan

Far Sense Kan also uses two Shinkan to tap the site, similar to Spring Finger Kan, but the Far Sense Kan taps only after needle is removed. Further, both Tapping Around Kan and Spring Finger Kan are versatile in their usage; they can be used for either tonifying or draining methods, but Far-Sense Kan is to be used only for the draining method: it taps the "opened" after-needled site (do not seal the point when the needle is removed) to disperse the Evil Ki around the site, and release the muscular tensions.

◎ Tapping Around Kan

●The Origin of the Name

The Japanese name of this jutsu is "Kou-kan", which literally means "tapping/drumming Kan." Similar to Spring Finger Kan, this jutsu is to tap the skin around the needling site. But for this jutsu, tapping rhythm is more like taiko-drumming, bouncing and springing rhythm.

●Main Effects

Alleviate the pain by dispersing the Evil Ki stagnated on site (reducing method).

●How to Hold a Shinkan

Use Sashi-de (needling hand). Place the index finger to press the tip of Shinkan, and hold it by the thumb and middle finger (the ring and small fingers support).

●Technique

Insert the needle at the targeted depth, and remove the Shinkan. Leave the Oshi-de (pushing hand) as well. Hold an empty Shinkan between the thumb, middle and index fingers. Tap the skin surrounding the needled site

Tapping Around Kan

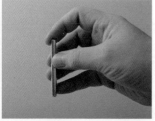

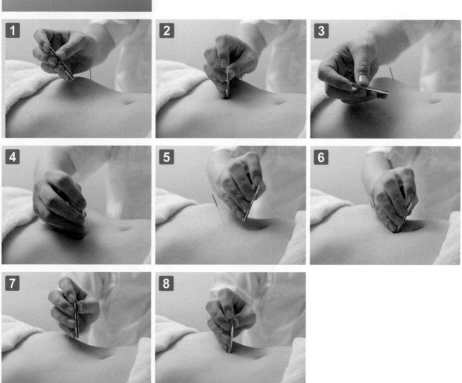

1. Insert the needle at the targeted depth, and remove the Shinkan. Takeaway the Oshi-de (pushing hand).
2. Hold the empty Shinkan by the thumb, the middle and index fingers of Sashi-de (needling hand).Tap the skin surrounding the needled site with a fine, fast rhythm.
3. Shift the Shinkan to nearby area
4. Tap again at the fine, fast rhythm
5. Move the Shinkan to another area
6. Tap again at the fine, fast rhythm
7. Continue till it covers all surrounding areas
8. Make sure the tapping rhythm is consistently fast and fine

with the fine, fast rhythm.

Shift the Shinkan and tap again, and continue till it covers all the surrounding areas you would like to influence. Feel Ki change underneath the skin.

When needling is shallow (the sites such as extremities or Jin-Well points), you may hold the needle lightly (so that the needle does not come off) while tapping the surrounding area.

•Clinical Usage Examples

- Alleviate the pain on the side of the head/face such as toothache and/or migraine by releasing the muscular tensions. Use TH20 (Jaosun) point, for example, to alleviate the side pain by using Tapping-Around Kan (reducing method).
- Contract common cold or flu and dislike the cold, use DU14 (DaZhui) point: needle on DU14 and tap the nape of the neck and rhomboid muscles (between the scapulae) to open the subcutaneous to promote sweating (reducing method)
- Alleviate the pain in the IT Band to the knee (which can be slightly bent) by needling GB39 (Xuanzhong) against the meridian flow, to release the tension in the external thigh muscles and the knee (tonifying method)
- For fullness and/or swelling of the abdomen, tonify the lower abdomen and use ST44 (NeiTing) and SP4 (Gongsun) (Induction).

◎ Spring Finger Kan

•the Origin of the Name

Similar to Tapping Around Kan in essence, but Spring Finger Kan jutsu uses both hands using two Shinkan to tap the surrounding areas of the needled site; so the tapping rhythm is stronger, more springy and bouncy.

Spring Finger Kan

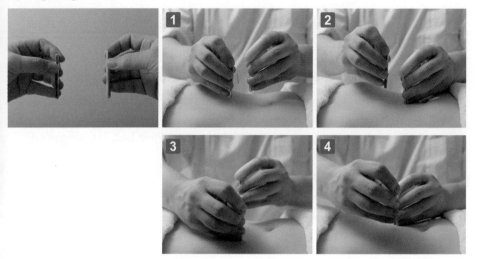

1. Once the needle is inserted at the targeted depth, remove the Shinkan. Each hand takes an empty Shinkan, held vertically.
2. Tap the surrounding area of the needled site, like drumming a taiko.
3. Tapping should be done alternatively, with a fast, light rhythm. Make sure to thoroughly cover the surrounding area.
4. The more taps given, the better.

●Main Effects

Disperse the Stagnation of Ki and/or Evil Heat (draining method)

Move Ki and Blood for better circulations (tonifying method)

●How to Hold a Shinkan

Both hands are used. Hold a Shinkan in each hand, like a small drumstick – your index fingers to be placed at the top of Shinkan, and thumb and middle to little fingers support holding the Shinkan vertically.

●Technique

Once the needle is inserted at the targeted depth, remove the Shinkan. Each hand takes an empty Shinkan. Hold vertically and tap the surrounding area of the needled site, like drumming a taiko. Tapping should come one at a time and alternatively, with a fast rhythm. The more taps given, the better. Similar to Tapping-Around Kan, but this jutsu use both hands

and two Shikan to give a faster, fine rhythm vibration. Feel Ki change underneath the skin.

●Clinical Usage Examples
- For shortness of breath and/or pressure in chest, use CV17 (Shanzhong), LU1 (Zhongfu) (draining method).
- For cold, numb legs that are difficult to move, use BL57 (Chengshan) (tonifying method).
- For abnormal vaginal bleeding, apply Tapping-Around justu to KD2 (Rangu), KD6 (Zhaohai), or KD10 (Yingu), and also apply the Spring-Finger Kan for GB39 (Xuanzhong) (induction).

◎ Far Sense Kan
●The Origin of the Name
This jutsu affects far beyond the area of the needling site by using both hands to tap to give stimulations. Also, taps the "opened" area (draining method) with Shinkan after the needle is removed.

●Main Effects
Release the tension around the needle removal areas (after the needle is removed) by dispersing the Evil Ki (draining method).

Alleviate the chronic pain for excess and/or deficient conditions.

●How to Hold a Shinkan
Use both hands. Each hand to hold a Shinkan vertically by the thumb, middle and ring fingers while the index finger to be on the top of the Shinkan.

●Technique
Far Sense Kan is the jutsu used after removing the needle. After applying draining needling method to the site, then right after the needle is removed, each hand holds an empty Shinkan vertically and taps the site. Tap one hand at a time, and tap different areas to thoroughly cover the sur-

Far Sense Kan

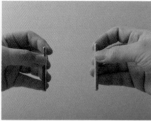

1. After applying reducing needling method to the site,
2. Remove the needle.
3. Each hand holds an empty Shinkan vertically, and taps the area of the site.
4. Tap one hand at a time, and alternatively.
5. Tap different areas to be thorough.
6. Make sure the tapping is a consistent rhythm

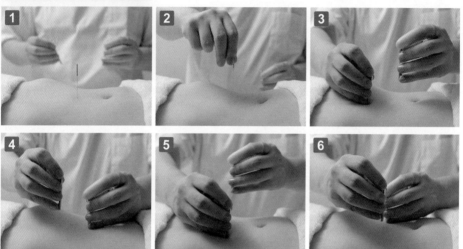

rounding area.

●Clinical Usage Example

- For leg pain especially joint pain with bone or tendon underline problems, apply for SP5 (Shangqiu) and KD6 (Zhaohai) (draining method).

◎ Muscle Rubbing Kan

●The Origin of the Name

Named Muscle Rubbing as it aims to gather and move Ki and Blood to the area by rubbing the muscles surrounding the needling site.

Muscle Rubbing Kan

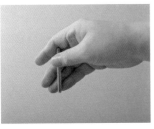

1. Once the needle is inserted at the targeted depth, remove the Shinkan. Hold the needle handle by the thumb and index finger of Oshi-de (pushing hand).
2. Sashi-de (needling hand) holds an empty Shinkan vertically and rubs and presses against the surrounding skin.
3. Follow the curvature of the body while rubbing and pressing.
4. Move smoothly in the surrounding area to cover the area thoroughly.
5. Make sure the Shinkan tip follows all the curvatures when moving around.

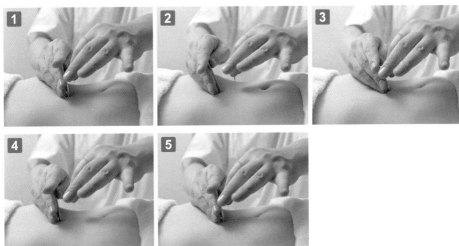

●Main Effect
Move Ki and Blood in the deficient, cold site (tonifying method).

●How to Hold a Shinkan
Similar to Tapping-Around Kan, place the index finger on the top of the Shinkan, and hold it by the thumb and middle, ring finger vertically.

●Technique
Once the needle is inserted at the desired depth, remove the Shinkan. Use Oshi-de (pushing hand) to hold the handle of the needle to stabilize. Use Sashi-de (needling hand) to hold an empty Shinkan vertically. Rub and press against the surrounding area by the tip of the Shinkan. Follow the curvature of the body for rubbing and pressing, and rub thoroughly.

●Clinical Usage Examples

- Alleviate abdominal pain due to Cold (male), Alleviate Okestu (Blood stagnation), Ki stagnation abdominal pain and/or reduce white vaginal discharge (female). For both genders, apply to the abdominal points (tonifying method).
- For upper body's paralysis, apply for TH5 (Waiguan) (draining method).

4. Needle Vibration Kan Jutsu

Dragon's Head Kan, Ingenious Dragon's Head Kan, Glowing Needle Kan, Internal Tuning Kan, Connecting Valley Kan

【 Main Effects 】
Strengthening the needling effects such as Hibiki, tonification or draining, induction as needed. Also, Hibiki to be spread to the surrounding area (propagation after the Ki arrives, spread calm and gentle Hibiki to the whole body for harmonizing Ki and Blood.

【 Clinical Applications 】
- Swelling and constricting the side abdomen / stomach by deficient Spleen and/or Stomach.
- Pain in the stomach with chill or fever, and low appetite.
- Cold Injury causing chill but no sweat.
- Water Stagnation in the stomach, swelling or bloating the abdomen with cold extremities.
- Cold lower abdomen and diarrhea.

【 Jutsu Classifications 】
① Give vibrations to the needle head (handle) horizontally: Dragon's Head, Ingenious Dragon's Head Kan and Glowing Needle Kan.
② Give vibrations by tapping the needle's holding hand (finger nails): Internal tuning Kan, Connecting valley Kan

●Dragon's Head Kan, Ingenious Dragon's Head Kan and Glowing Needle Kan

They are similar in their objectives in general, to give vibrations to the needling site. The main difference is that the Dragon' Head Kan taps with one Shinkan, using one hand, while Ingenious Dragon's Head Kan taps with two Shikan using both hands. The Glowing Needle Kan technique looks different from the two jutsu, as the Shinkan gives pendulum swings to the needle vibrations.

●Internal Tuning Kan and Connecting Valley Kan

They are also similar in their objectives and techniques. The main difference between them is that the Internal Tuning Kan taps the fingernail of the Oshi-de (pushing hand), and the Connecting Valley Kan taps the needle handle.

Further, Internal Tuning Kan is often used with deep needling, and used in each step while needling depth goes deeper: for example, this jutsu is applied 2-3 times while needling depth goes deeper step by step (similar to Raising Sun Kan).

◎ Dragon's Head Kan

●The Origin of the Name

The acupuncture needle handle part is often called the Dragon's Head, and this jutsu gives vibrations to the side of the Dragon's Head.

●Main Effects

Support Hibiki , arrival of Ki (Hibiki)
Induce Ki to the extremities of the Meridian (induction)

●How to Hold a Shinkan

Use Sashi-de (needling hand) only. An empty Shinkan to be held by

Dragon's Head Kan

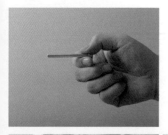

1. Once the needle is inserted at the targeted depth, remove the Shinkan and Oshi-de (pushing hand).Hold on to an empty Shinkan at the right side of the needle.
2. Tap the right side of the Dragon's Head (needle head) .
3. Needle to vibrate finely (left – right) .
4. Tap the left side of the Dragon's Head (needle head) .
5. Needle to vibrate finely, same as #3 .
6. Give sufficient vibrations from both sides.

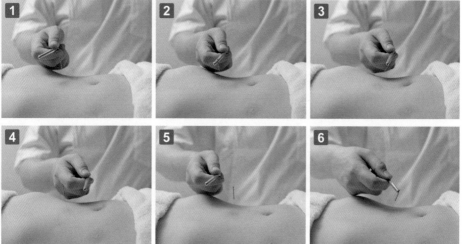

Note: For shallow needling, use Oshi-de (pushing hand) gently holds the needle while tapping. Repeat until giving sufficient vibrations. (The needle is supposed to finely move left to right, or right or left, while tapping.)

the thumb and index fingers horizontally.

●Technique

Once the needle is inserted at the targetted depth, remove both the Shinkan and Oshi-de (pushing hand). The thumb and index finger of Sashi-de (needling hand) holds an empty Shinkan horizontally. Give a tap on the side of the Dragon's Head (needle head) to give fine vibrations to the needle. Tap from right side, move to the left side.

For shallow needling, use Oshi-de (pushing hand) to gently hold the needle while tapping. Repeat until given sufficient vibrations until Ki is changed. (The needle is supposed to finely move left to right, or right left, while tapping.)

●Clinical Usage Examples
- When swelling or pain caused by deficient Spleen and/or Stomach, apply for LV13 (Zhangmen) (Hibiki) and/or PC6 (Neiguan) (induction)
- When the wrist is swelling and stiff, apply for PC7 (Daling) (Harmonization)
- When the palm is warm and stiff and painful, apply for PC6 (Neiguan) (Induction)
- When the throat is sore and painful, apply for LI7 (Wenliu) (induction).
- For acute watery diarrhea with deficient conditions, first to tonify and warm the abdomen, then apply for KD7 (Fuliu) (harmonization).

◎ Ingenious Dragon's Head Kan

●The Origin of the Name
Similar to the Dragon's Head Kan, but this jutsu uses both hands using two Shinkan to tap the Dragon's Head "crafty," "skillfully" and "ingeniously" - to give fine vibrations.

●Main Effects
Support Hibiki / Ki arrival (HIbiki)
Harmonize Ki and Blood after the Ki arrival (harmonization)

●How to Hold a Shinkan
Use both hands. Each hand holds an empty Shinkan horizontally by the thumb and index fingers.

●Technique
Once the needle is inserted at the targeted depth, remove Shinkan and Oshi-de (pushing hand). Each hand's thumb and index finger hold an empty Shinkan horizontally, then tap the side of the Dragon's Head (needle handle) with each Shinkan. Tap alternatively from the right and left

Ingenious Dragon's Head Kan

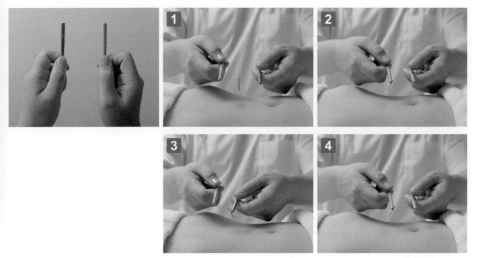

1. Once the needle is inserted at the targeted depth, remove Shinkan and Oshi-de (pushing hand). Each hand's thumb and index finger holds an empty Shinkan horizontally.
2. Tap the right side of the Dragon's Head (needle handle).
3. Tap the left side.
4. Tap alternately from the right and left side with a fine, fast rhythm. Repeat until given sufficient vibrations.

side with a fine, fast rhythm. Repeat until given sufficient vibrations.
(The needle is supposed to finely move left to right or right or left while tapping.)

●Clinical Usage Examples
- For elbow muscle or tendon pain, apply to LU5 (Chize), LI11 (Quchi) and PC3 (Quze) (harmonization)
- For the pain alongside the knee and inner thigh or hip joint, apply for GB31 (Fengshi) (harmonization).

◎ Glowing Needle Kan

•The Origin of the Name

The Shinkan gives vibrations to the needles via a pendulum swing movement: it reflects light during the swings to give a shiny glow. Hence it was named as Glowing Needle Kan Jutsu.

•Main effects

Promote Hibiki, the arrival of Ki (Hibiki)

Encourage the Hibiki to the surrounding area (propagation)

•How to Hold a Shinkan

Use Sashi-de (needling hand) only. Hold the tip of an empty Shinkan by the tips of the thumb and index finger, like holding a pendulum.

Glowing Needle Kan

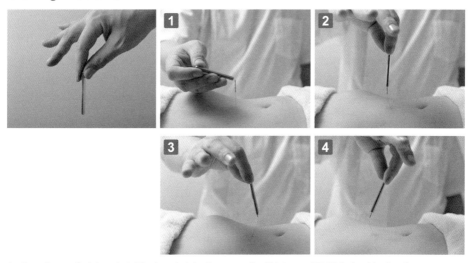

1. Once the needle is inserted at the targeted depth, remove the Shinkan and Oshi-de (pushing hand).
2. Place a Shinkan back to the inserted needle half way.
3. Hold the tip of the Shinkan to give pendulum swings to the left.
4. Pendulum swing to the right – continue alternating until sufficient swings have been given.

●Technique

Once the needle is inserted at the targeted depth, remove the Shinkan and Oshi-de (pushing hand). Make sure the needle is stable. Place a Shinkan halfway over the inserted needle. Then hold the tip of the Shinkan to give pendulum swings (right to left rather than a full circle motion). Repeat until given sufficient vibrations.

●Clinical Usage Examples

- For swelling and painful legs, apply for ST35(Xiyan) and/or Medial Xiyan (Hibiki).
- For chronic cough with long-term illness and/or decreased physical strength, apply for the SanJao (Triple Heater) Meridian points (propagation).

◎ Internal Tuning Kan

●the Origin of the Name

It is named as Internal Tuning Kan as this jutsu harmonizes and tunes the deeper layers of the body (subcutaneous, vessels, muscles and bones). As the needle insertion is deepened, the stimulation goes deeper.

●Main Effects

Disperse Ki, Food, Water or Blood stagnation (draining method).

Induce Ki to the extremities or Jin-Well points of the meridians (induction).

●How to Hold a Shinkan

Use Sashi-de (needling hand). Hold an empty Shinkan horizontally and rather loosely with the thumb and index finger.

●Technique

Once the needle is inserted to around 4-5mm depth, make sure the Oshi-de (pushing hand) stabilizes the needle by the thumb and the index fingertips. Hold an empty Shinkan with the Sashi-de (needling

73

Internal Tuning Kan

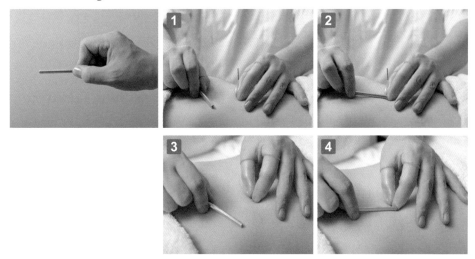

1. Once the needle is inserted to around 4-5mm depth, make sure the Oshi-de (pushing hand) stabilizes the needle between the thumb and the index finger tips. Hold an empty Shinkan by the Sashi-de (needling hand).
2. Hold the Shinkan horizontally and use it to tap the fingernails that are holding the needle.
3. Repeat tapping with consistent force and rhythm.
4. When complete, pause to tap, deepen the needle insertion for about another 5mm. Then, the Shinkan taps the fingertips again.
   Note: when removing the needle, reverse these steps (pull about 5mm and tap, and pull and tap). This jutsu is commonly used for the sites such as the abdomen where needles can be inserted deeper. But it can be used for other sites such as extremities where only needle insertion and tapping is needed.

hand) horizontally and tap the fingernails that are holding the needle. Once finished, deepen the needle insertion for about another 5mm. Then, the Shinkan taps the fingertips again.

When removing the needle, reverse these steps (pull about 4-5mm and tap, and pull and tap). This jutsu is commonly used for sites such as the abdomen where needles can be inserted deeper, but it can be used for other sites such as the extremities which need fewer steps.

●Clinical Usage Examples
- For hiccups related to upper abdomen Water stagnation, use CV12 (Zhongwan) to disperse the Water stagnation and move Ki and Blood in the upper, middle abdomen (draining method).

- For lower abdomen pain by gas and/or bowel stagnation, use ST29 (Guilai) to move the bowel movement and alleviate pain (draining method).
- For joint pain, use LI4 (Hegu), ST36 (Zhusanli), BL40 (Weizhong), TH4 (Yangchi) and BL11 (Dazhui) for shallow insertion using two-step needle insertion (draining method).
- For common cold/flu related headache, fever, first tonify the abdomen and disperse the nape of the neck, apply this jutsu for BL40 (Weizhong) to induce upper body pain to the lower body to harmonize the whole body (induction).
- For constipation, first needle on the lower abdomen, then apply this jutsu for ST36 (Zhusanli) to move bowel down (induction).

◎ Connecting Valley Kan

●The Origin of the Name

This justu was named as Connecting Valley Kan as it was originally used to move Ki through the "valley" which is a small "dent" space such as between the joints and bones.

●Main Effect

Alleviate pain in legs, knees or foot where Ki or Blood are injured and deficient by moving the Ki and Blood (tonifying method).

●How to Hold the Shinkan

Use Oshi-de (pushing hand). Hold the Shinkan horizonally by the thumb and index finger.

●Technique

Once the needle is inserted at the targeted depth, remove the Shinkan. Hold the needle by the thumb and index finger of Oshi-de (pushing hand) to stabilize. Sashi-de (needling hand) holds an empty Shinkan horizontally, next to the needle. Tap fast the needle handle by Shinkan from the oblique upper angle. Tap light and fast to make the needle vibrate.

Connecting Valley Kan

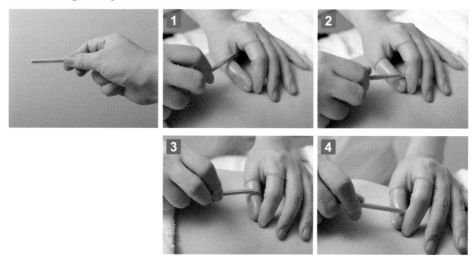

1. Once the needle is inserted at the targeted depth, remove the Shinkan. Hold just below the needle handle by the thumb and index finger of Oshi-de (pushing hand). Sashi-de (needling hand) holds an empty Shinkan.
2. Tap the needle handle with the Shinkan to make the needle vibrate.
3. Make sure to have the Shinkan repeat tapping with consistent force and rhythm.
4. Keep tapping to make the needle vibrate.

●Clinical Usage Examples

    -    For cramping and painful legs, use ST41 (Jiexi), GB42 (Diwuhui) and BL62 (Shenmai). They are called "Leg's Three Corner Points"(tonifying method).

    -    For common cold/flu fever and aversion to cold, needle shallowly DU14 (Dazhui) and surrounding area and apply this jutsu to promote sweating (tonifying method).

Chapter 6

Waichi Sugiyama, Founder of "Kanshin Method"

Father of Japanese Acupuncture

If you are an acupuncturist and use "Shinkan (guide tube)" clinically, you might want to know about Kengyo Waichi Sugiyama. The reason is that the use of Shinkan in acupuncture treatment, the "Kan Shin Method" was established and spread all over Japan by Waichi in the seventeenth century.

Kengyo was the highest ranking of blind/visually impaired official in the medieval and pre-modern times in Japan, they specialized in medicine such as acupuncture, Anma or music fields.

Waichi Sugiyama is recognized as one of the most distinguished Kengyo officials in Japan. He established and spread the Kanshin Method of acupuncture. He is also known as a personal doctor for Tsunayoshi Tokugawa, the fifth Shogun of the Tokugawa Shogunate. Further, Waichi Sugiyama is known and respected overseas, he is called the "Father of Japanese Acupuncture"

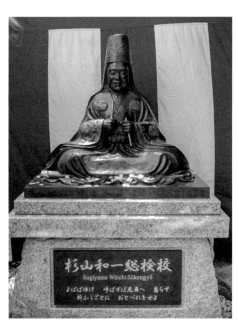

As he was born and lived about 400 years ago, there are more than a few uncertrain events in his life. Hence, this book introduces the life of Waichi Sugiyama. With the co-operation of Mr. Jikan Oura,one of the first researchers of Waichi Sugiyama, it is as close to truth of the historical facts as possible.

The statue of Waichi at Enoshima Shrine

Childhood: Aspired to be an Acupuncture Doctor acupuncture doctor

Waichi Sugiyama was born as the first boy in the middle-class Samurai family of Shigemasa Sugiyama, in Tsu city, Ise province (current Mie prefecture), which is located in the west region of main island of Japan. He was born healthy; however, at a young age he lost his vision from an infective disease, assumed to be measles. The age he lost his vision was said to be 5 or 10 years old.

Around this time, the occupations for the visually impaired people were generally limited to becoming either a biwa (Japanese lute) playing minstrel, or a practitioner of Anma massage which was called "Kneading Treatment." Waichi's mother had him learn the biwa instrument, but he did not want to become a biwa player.

When he became 16, he told his parents that he wanted to become an acupuncture doctor. Waichi was a gentle boy, he wanted to be a doctor to save people rather than a samurai who kill each other, as he had witnessed while he still had his vision.

Aiming to be an acupuncture doctor was a hard choice. It required a very strong will for the visually impaired person like Waichi. In fact, at that time there were only three blind acupuncture doctors in Japan (Takuichi Yamase, Jokan Yamakawa, and Josen Iwafune). As Waichi's determination was firm, his father Shigemasa eventually understood and decided to support his son's will.

Around this time, acupuncture medicine could only be learned in big cities like Kyoto or Edo (current Tokyo). Normally visually impaired people acquired knowledge through visually impaired people, but there were no blind acupuncture doctors in Kyoto, which is closer to Ise province where Waichi lived. Then Shigemasa, Waichi's father found Takuichi Yamase in Edo. Shigemasa ased if Waichi could become an apprentice for Takuichi, and it was accepted. Become an apprentice for Takuichi, and it was accepted. In 1626, Waichi moved to Edo with a servant. He was 17 years old.

Takuichi Yamase taught mostly Anma for the first three years (1626-1630) to Waichi. At that time, Anma was called "Kneading Treatment," and treatment was done by skillful hands. Takuihi intended to let Waichi acquire deep understanding of the human body anatomy by using his hands. This would be an essential skill for visually impaired people to practice medicine. Waichi passionately practiced Kneading Treatment, and his techniques steadily improved.

After three years passed, Waichi mastered Kneading Treatment techniques. Then Takuichi started teaching acupuncture jutsu (techniques). However, Waichi had to face an unexpected failure. He had to discontinue the practice of acupuncture. There is a theory that Waichi was lazy and not sharp enough to acquire the acupuncture techniques, and was eventually expelled. However, in order to know the true reason behind this event, it is important to understand the historical background about how acupuncture was taught around this era in Japan.

Around this time in Japanese acupuncture, there was not enough textbooks to learn from, the subject was largely taught verbally by masters using very simple illustrations of acupuncture channels and points. Hence, there were many cases of malpractice and in some cases, patients died from the wrong treatment. Moreover, as visually impaired, both Takuichi and Waichi could not see such illustrations.

Moreover, at that time the major needling method was the "Nen Shin Method" which used long, thick needles (thicker than 0.34mm diameter, the Chinese gage 28 or less), directly needling into the skin while twisted between thumb and index fingers. The stimulation of the insertion is very strong, there were cases when patients lost consciousness, or even lost life from it. Around this time, acupuncture doctors needed to master the "Reverse Needling" technique how to revive consciousness for the patients who passed out from strong needling stimulation. Medical accidents and malpractices were often associated with acupuncture medicine around this time.

Waichi was known to be a gentle soul. He could not accept the possibility that he may cause death to his patient due to a needling accident. That was the main reason Waichi could not continue practicing

acupuncture medicine further. It was the time when 3 years passed after Waichi started his apprenticeship for Takuichi Yamase. Waichi was only 20 years old at that time, and his soul was young and gentle. However, Takuichi had to stop teaching Waichi if he could not learn "Nen Shin Method" needling and proceed to acquire further skills. Takuichi had to be feeling devasted to expel Waichi who was diligently practicing Anma for the last 3 years in order to become an acupuncture doctor, but eventually, Waichi was expelled by Takuichi.

Revelation of God

Giving up his path to become an acupuncture doctor means he could become a biwa minstrel – or simply die in despair. He could not give up the idea of becoming an acupuncture doctor. He became desperate and decided to make a pilgrimage to the Benzaiten God in Enoshima island. Built as a shrine in the cave by an imperial order of the Emperor Kinmei (around A.D. 510 - 571), the Benzaiten god was known as the most respected spiritual place in the Kanto district of Japan. The shrine consists of two caves, the "upper shrine" was 152m deep, and "lower shrine" was 56m deep, both of which were made from coastal erosion. The practice to

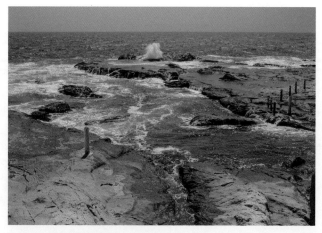

The sea at Enoshima island

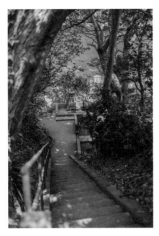

Current Enoshima steps (Kanagawa, Japan)

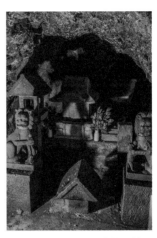

The original shrine of Enoshima Shrine (Kanagawa, Japan)

get a revelation was called "Okomori" which is to stay inside of the shrine cave without food for days to worship the God. Saint Kobo, Saint Nichiren were known to practice at Benzaiten. This fasting practice was known to be unforgiving as no food was allowed, just water. Many people died during the practice. The readiness to die was required if there is no revelation of God during "Okomori." Waichi, therefore, went to Enoshima Island with a determination to obtain a revelation from God, he accepted a possibility of losing his life for it.

The revelation of God Waichi was willing to sacrifice his life for, was prevention of medical accident in acupuncture. Waichi desperately needed a more secure way to practice acupuncture medicine for him to continue studying, he thought further healthy development was needed for acupuncture medicine. Waichi arrived at Enoshima island with his servant Kiyosuke, and he started his stay in the lower shrine cave. At this time, Benzaiten's "Okomori" was practiced for seven days as one cycle. Waichi completed his first seven days of fasting and praying, while enduring severe coldness and hunger. He did not obtain any revelation of God. He continued another seven days of fasting and praying to God, but he saw nothing coming. In this "Okomori" practice, many people lost their lives around 10 days, so surviving 14 days was miraculous enough, but Waichi kept going for another seven days of fasting and praying.

Then, Benzaiten God, who Waichi prayed with his life, suddenly appeared to him and gave him a heavenly ethereal idea that he "will use a tube-like supportive tool for easier, safer needling." This revelation of God, which finally came to Waichi at the risk of his own life, was the beginning of the birth of Kanshin needling method.

In other words, the historical truth of the birth of Kanshin Method which we acupuncturists practice in our daily clinical practice, is actually the gift Waichi received at the risk of his life by sincerely wishing to know how to prevent the acupuncture medical accident.

Establishing Kanshin Method in Kyoto

It was recorded that Waichi returned to Edo to be with Takuichi Yamase, after finishing this fasting practice in Enoshima island where he received the voice from Benzaiten God. Waichi reported to Takuichi that he received the idea to use "Shinkan" (guide tube) as a result of fasting. Waichi stayed with Takuichi another 5 years (1630 – 1635) to learn acupuncture despite him already being expelled. It is considered that Takuichi understood and supported the idea of Kanshin method brought back by Waichi.

After 5 years had passed, Takuichi recommended Waichi move to Kyoto where acupuncture was used more commonly, and the standard was higher. Indeed, Kyoto was "the place to be" for competitive acupuncture doctors and there was more information about acupuncture. Kyoto was also a mecca of acupuncture needle craftmanship, there were more high-level technicians and more advanced manufacturing technologies available. As there are far more shrines and temples which need highly sophisticated metal manufacturing, Kyoto was considered the most advanced level in metal craftmanship. Acupuncture needles are so thin and refined they require such high level of metal manufacturing technology, and Waichi needed these in order to elaborate his "Kanshin Method," as well as for him to acquire a higher level of knowledge and skill. Takuichi Manase knew about Kyoto's competitive environment, as he himself learned from Yoshiaki Irie who established "Irie Style" in Kyoto.

Because of his own experience, Takuichi recommended Waichi to move to Kyoto to learn "Irie Style" acupuncture. However, Yoshiaki Irie, the master of Takuichi was already deceased. Takuichi wrote a letter to Toyoaki, the son of Yoshiaki, asking to let Waichi learn Irie Style under Yoshiaki. Thanks to Takuichi's effort, Waichi was accepted by Yoshiaki Irie, and left for Kyoto in 1635.

In Kyoto, acupuncture medicine was far more commonly used than in Edo at that time. Besides "Irie Style," there were more than a few other styles such as "Mosonomura Style," "Suruga Style," and "Mubun Style" and "Myoshin Style." Waichi learned "Irie Style" under Toyoaki Irie, as planned. As for the needling method used at this time, there was an acupuncture needling method which used a tube called "Zudan-gake" (it is assumed this tube was made from bamboo tree). Hence, it was not exactly the case that Waichi was the first person to use a tube for acupuncture needle insertion. But it is the fact that Waichi Sugiyama was the first person who invented a metal tube used for acupuncture needle insertion and he spread this method all over Japan.

Around this time, Waichi was able to access some classic medical textbooks from China that were not available in Edo, such as "Su Wen." "Spiritual Pivot," "NanJing," etc. He read these books while he was studying at the Irie family for the next 7 years until 1642. After he spent 7 years, he stayed 3 more years in Kyoto until 1645, studying further with Chishin Tanaka, the first apprentice of Joshitsu Matsuzawa who founded the "Myo Shin Style." Waichi is also thought to have studied "Henju ken kei an" who is considered to be a female due to her writing style (Note: at that time, anomalous cursive syllabary writing style was used by females). She was considered to be the author of the book called "Shinkyu Daiwabun" (can be translated as "Acupuncture and Moxibustion in Japan") which will be addressed later. Also, in Kyoto, there was another popular needling method called "Dashin jutsu", which was spread by Isai Misono who founded the Misono Style. This Dashin jutsu (tapping needling jutsu) is not widely known anymore, but needles are inserted by tapping with a small wooden mallet. However, this method was not used by Irie Style where Waichi learned, but its unique "tapping the handle of the needles"

insertion method seemed to be similar to Kanshin Method, created by Waichi. There is a possibility he learned this method and incorporated it into his technique, in order to elaborate his Kanshin Method.

While spending time in Kyoto, Waichi kept learning, and after numerous trials and errors, he eventually invented a metal-made Shinkan (guide tube) to establish his unique, innovative Kanshin Method needling. Waichi also created many techniques /jutsu to give additional stimulations on the acupuncture sites by using the guide tube itself. These techniques/jutsu are called "Fourteen Kan Jutsu."

Compiled Acupuncture Textbooks

Kanshin Method made acupuncture needling safer and easier. Further, this method became a foundation of "another historical achievement" Waichi Sugiyama accomplished in his life. At this time, common needling techniques such as Nen-shin (from China) or Dashin methods all required the use of thicker diameter needles (assumed to be more than 0.34mm). On the other hand, Kanshin Method is a guide-tube method allows much thinner (0.20mm or less) diameter needles to be used. Thinner diameter needles without using guide tube, can easily bend when being inserted into skin. But by using a guide tube, these thinner needles do not bend and are inserted smoothly. Waichi also devoted his time to develop thinner acupuncture needles during his stay in Kyoto. Without using the guide tube, it is difficult to use thinner needles for acupuncture, so we can say the thinner needles are the creation of Waichi who invented the guide tubes. Overseas eastern medicine experts commonly say the use of thinner needles and guide tube (Shinkan) are the major characteristics of Japanese style acupuncture. Therefore, we can say that Japanese acupuncture was shaped by Waichi Sugiyama.

Waichi envisioned to return to Edo to improve the quality of the acupuncture education for the visually impaired population, so that it could be a safer and more stable occupation for the visually impaired people. He was preparing to achieve this goal while working on thinner needles and Shinkan development in Kyoto. He organized the newly acquired knowledge

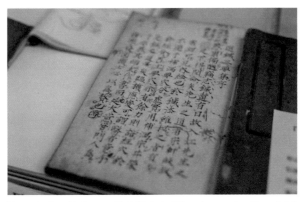

The book "Senshin Sanyou Shu" ("Selected Three Acupuncture Essentials")
edited by Waichi

in acupuncture medicine in Kyoto, and started writing the textbooks for teaching acupuncture. As stated previously, when Waichi was apprenticing to Takuichi Yamase, there were many acupuncture accidents and mistakes coming from the lack of solid teaching with textbooks. He thought the occupation itself might face a risk of decline without such improvements. Waichi felt the strong need of improvements of safety and education of acupuncture by his own hard experience from his own apprenticeship. He was known to have a caring heart. He must have felt that visually impaired people who wish to be acupuncture physicians should not go through the same hardships he experienced.

There are acupuncture textbooks called "Ryo-ji no Daigai Shu" (can be translated as "Major Outlines of Remedies and Treatments") which is a trilogy editted by Waichi. He also was involved in a book in two volumes called "Senshin Sanyou Shu" (can be translated as "Selected Three Acupuncture Essentials") and also "Igaku Setsuyo Shu" (can be translated as "Dictionary of Medical Terms"). Waichi's published work is referred to as "Sugiyama Ryu Sambu Sho" ("Three Books of the Sugiyama Style") which is a collection of the foundations of acupuncture medical theories. Recent studies found that Waichi himself wrote the "Senshin Sanyou Shu," however, "Ryo-ji no Daigai Shu" was the re-edit using the Chinese characters and Hiragana (Japanese cursive syllabary) combined, of the original book "Shinkyu Daiwabun" written by Henju-ken-kei-an, who

used anomalous cursive syllabary writing style. It is also understood now that the "Igaku Setsuyo Shu" was published after Waichi's death, edited based on Waichi's lectures, by Yasuichi Miura, a successor Kengyo and an apprentice of Waichi.

Around the time when Waichi spent his 10 years in Kyoto, Toyoaki Irie passed away. Called upon on the verge of death, Waichi was left with his will saying "you must hand the acupuncture treatment down to posterity." After that, Waichi returned to Edo to realize his master's will and to achieve his own goals. In Edo, Waichi opened a private clinic to start practicing while taking apprentices of his own by opening a private school in Kojimachi (current Chiyoda-ward). With his high capacity, coming from his thorough training in Kyoto, the mecca for acupuncture, his clinic was immediately packed by patients and many apprentices followed. Waichi started teaching what he learned in Kyoto as well as Kanshin Method techniques. Around his time, acupuncture techniques were mainly taught secretly as a family tradition, so Waichi innovated by sharing his skills publicly, and accepting his apprentices proactively by opening a school.

Shogunate's Physician and "Sugiyama Shin Den Ryu"

In 1670, Waichi became Kengyo at age 61. The reputation of Waichi Sugiyama as an acupuncture doctor spread further in Edo and eventually was heard by the Edo Castle. In 1680, Waichi was given an audience by the fifth Shogunate Tsunayoshi (Tokugawa) to give treatment to his chronic disease. Then, Waichi continued treating Tsunayoshi. By 1685, he became a court physician and was bestowed with the house in Dosan-Gashi inside of the Tokiwabashi Bridge (within the Edo Castle). Tsunayoshi's chronic condition was called as "lingering disease," (bura-bura yamai) which was speculated to be a type of neurosis. As Tsunayoshi was in the position to receive strong stress, there is no surprise he was suffering from stress-induced conditions.

In 1682, Waichi's private school was recognized by the Tokugawa

Shogunate, and newly opened in Ogawa-machi as "Acupuncture Treatment School" for the visually impaired. The world's first school for the visually impaired people was opened by Valentin Haüy in Paris, France in 1784. Before that, education for visually impaired was done individually, but Valentin Haüy elevated it to become a public group education. On the other hand, Acupuncture Treatment School by Waichi Sugiyama was opened in 1682, nearly 100 years prior to Valentin Haüy, so the first school for the visually impaired was actually this Acupuncture Treatment School by Waichi Sugiyama.

The Acupuncture Treatment School received support from Tokugawa Shogunate, and was told to educate either visually impaired or sighted, in order to continue the acupuncture profession. The Tokugawa Shogunate promised job support for those who were trained thoroughly and diligently. Waichi, as a Kengyo, encourgaed people who wanted to be trained as acupuncture physicians, to join his acupuncture school for proper study and training. Each individual would have a ranking depending on their level of understanding and skills. He later regulated that acupuncture was to be administrated by those who were licensed from the acupuncture schools.

With these efforts, acupuncture education standard was dramatically improved, and acupuncture treatment was established as a safe medicine. Acupuncture and Anma professions were recognized as an occupation for the visually impaired. There were a number of apprentices from Waichi' school who became medical officers for the government.

Further, Waichi Sugiyama was appointed by the fifth Shogun Tsunayoshi Tokugawa, to become a "Sokengyo" (the highest ranking of Kengyo), to lead the "Tou Dou Za" which is the national support group among visually impaired men, established in the 860s.

One of the revenue sources of Tou Dou Za was lending money. This financial business was supported by various protective policies by the Tokugawa Shogunate. However, many people took advantages of such policies and made a profit out of it, and Tou Dou Za was gradually rotting from within by this vice financial business. Tsunayoshi wanted to reverse the situation, and appointed Waichi as Sokengyo to lead reform of the Tou

Dou Za regulations. This Sokengyo, the highest ranking Kengyo position, was a newly created position for Waichi by Shogun Tsunayoshi. It was considered that Tsunayoshi fully trusted Waichi not only as an acupuncture physician, but also as a council with his ability and personality.

Therapist often acts as a personal counselor for the patient, and the ability for giving personal advice is especially important for neurosis like Tsunayoshi's case. Waichi gradually became a personal consultant for Tsunayoshi through his acupuncture treat-

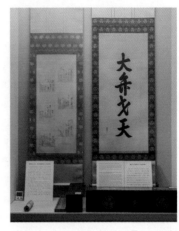

A big hanging scroll given by Tsunayoshi Tokugawa Shognate

ment. It was thought that there was a trust between them, possibly like a father and the son. Tsunayoshi was 46 years old and Waichi was 82 years old.

The next year, June 18th in 1693, Waichi was bestowed a large amount of land (about 8,925 square meters) and a town house in the area called "One Eye" in Honjo (current Sumida-ku, Tokyo). Town houses, in Japan around that time were common housing complexes, so Waichi could gain the rent as his revenue. Further, Tsunayoshi was concerned about old Waichi still regularly visiting Benzaiten in Enoshima Island which was far away. So Tsunayoshi asked for a special arrangement called Bunrei, which was to share the spirit of sacred Benzaiten God in the original Enoshima Island to Honjo at Waichi's place so he did not have to make a trip. Tsunayoshi Shogun himself called the head of local shrine cave and asked him to give up the gold Benzaiten statue which was stored in Enoshima island, and had originated from Taira family (since Kamakura period in the fourteen century) and in return, gave the special status to the shrine to guarantee it would not pay tax in the future. June 18th in 1693, Tsunayoshi formally gave the statue to Waichi, and told him he did not have to make a long trip any more. This is an anecdote of how Tsunayoshi was connected and concerned deeply about Waichi.

Waichi, from Honjo One Eye place, rebuilt the Tou Do Za system by

implementing a big reorganization. By his efforts, Tou Do Za was repositioned to be a healthy professional support group for visually impaired people. Waichi contributed a lot to the visually impaired people, not only as an acupuncture physician and teacher of acupuncture medicine, but also for the welfare of them as a Sokengyo in politics.

In the same year, he was appointed to become "Gon Daisozu" a high-ranking chief priest, and allowed to wear scarlet red with a white surplice. However, with all his accomplishments, Waichi Sugiyama was neve been appointed to be a formal Shogunate physician for the whole Tokugawa family. Waichi was thought to be more of a personal doctor or counsel for the fifth Shogunate Tsunayoshi, rather than the doctor for the Edo Shogunate body.

In the following year in 1694, a magnificent shrine called "Honjo One Eye Benten Shrine" was built in the land owned by Waichi. The One Eye Benten Shrine immediately became a noted place in Edo, it gained a lot of respect from the common people of Edo. This shrine became a famous place and even added to the famous topography book called "Edo Meisho Zue" (translated as "the geography book of Edo's noted historical sites"). Many people, even people from O-oku (a chamber of the Shogunate inner palace) visited by boat. This shrine is currently called "Ejima Sugiyama Shrine" located in Ryogoku, Sumida-ku, Tokyo.

He passed away right after the establishment of One Eye Benten Shrine. His last moment was told as if he was falling asleep. He was 85 years old. The corpse was buried in Shimono-miya, Eno-shima in Kanagawa prefecture.

After his death, Yasuichi Miura became the leader of the Sugiyama Style and Waichi's teaching was spread further in Japan. Waichi's acupuncture school was opened at 45 places in Kanto. The Kanshin Method invented by Waichi, with his own verbal instruction, were further organized by the second generation Yasuichi Miura and the third generation Wadaichi Shimaura to become well-organized instruction books, called "Sugiyama Shin Den Ryu" (can be translated as "Sugiyama Style True Tradition").

Chapter 7

Waichi Sugiyama's Spirit

Major Attraction in Edo

After working many years for the Tsunayoshi Tokugawa Shognate, Sugiyama Waichi was bestowed with a large land (about 8,925 square meters) and a town house called "One Eye Mansion."

Waichi created a shrine to pray to Benzaiten at his own place. This magnificent shrine "Honjo One Eye Benten Shrine" (Note: Benten is a short name for Benzaiten) immediately became a noted place in Edo. Waichi's story had gained a lot of respect from the common people of Edo. This shrine became a famous place and was even added to the famous topography book called "Edo Meisho Zu e" (translated as "The Geography Book of Edo's Noted Historical Sites," a famous compilation at the end of Edo era) and many people, even people from O-oku ("the big interior" a chamber of the Shogunate inner palace) visited by boat. This shrine is currently called "Ejima Sugiyama Shrine" is located in Ryogoku, Sumida-ku, Tokyo.

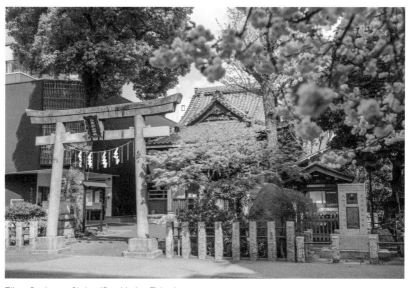

Ejima-Sugiyama Shrine (Sumida-ku, Tokyo)

After Waichi passed away, his apprentices built a resting place for his spirit in Honjo One Eye Benten Shrine, and enshrined Waichi's spirit as "Sokumyou-an Hermitage." Then time changed, in 1871, To-Do-Za, a national support group among visually impaired men, was eventually abolished. Originally established in the 860s, Waichi had

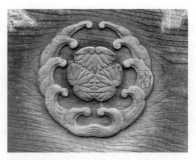

The Shrine Crest

worked for the group. Then in 1890, Honjo One Eye Benten Shrine was renamed as "Ejima Shrine." There was a "Sugiyama Shrine" which enshrined Waichi's spirit, created within the Ejima Shrine premises.

In 1923, Great Kanto Earthquake destroyed both Shrine palaces. They were rebuilt, then destroyed again during World War II. In 1952, the palace was rebuilt again: this time, these two shrines were merged into one shrine. The shrine was named as "Ejima Sugiyama Shrine."

Current Shrine represents two spirits: one is Waichi Sugiyama, and another one is called Ichikishimahime-no-mikoto. A goddess from Japanese mythology, identical to the Benzaizen who Waichi worshipped, which we explain in more detail later. The Mikoshi-ko (a storage for portable shrine) and offertory box are designed with the unique symbol of Ejima Sugiyama Shrine, which is a combination of ripples from Enoshima Island and the hollyhock-kamon (crest) which came from Tsunayoshi Tokugawa Shogunate.

The Precincts of Ejima Sugiyama Shrine

◎ A Palace

In the newly built palace after the World War II, you can see the original palace built in 1693 through the drawing "One Eye Benten" by Shoun Yamamoto, a famous Japanese painter (1870 - 1965), which is shown when entering into the sanctum of the palace.

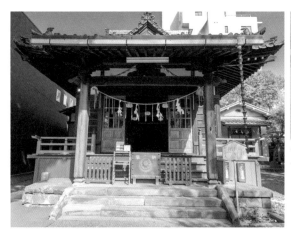
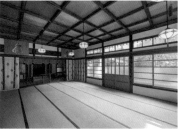

The Shrine palace (outside)
The Shrine palace (inside)

◎ The Cave

Within the precincts, there is "the cave" created in 1774 to show where Waichi stayed to obtain the revelation of Kanshin Method from the spirit of Bentenzai. This cave is much smaller than the actual one in Enoshima Island, and there is a stone statue of Waichi in front of the T-junction inside the cave. Waichi's statue was worshipped with others, including the god Ugajin, and the three goddess of wealth called Munakata Three Goddesses, which will be explained later.

This cave was renovated in 1793 and was not affected by the Great Kanto Earthquake, but the World War II fire made a huge crack in the ceiling, so it was rebuilt with reinforced-concrete to protect from any hazards, and the height of the whole shrine became taller because of this change. Within the cave, you can place a food offering to the white snake, which is known as a messenger for the Bentenzai God.

◎ Sugita Inari Shrine*

There is a small Inari Shrine in the Ejima Sugiyama Shrine called Sugita Inari Shrine. It has been there since old time, and no one knows who created it nor who it enshrines.

*Inari Shrine is dedicated to a god who looks after the grain.

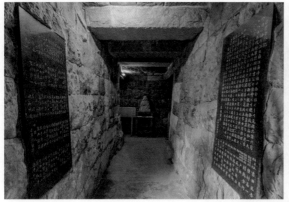

The cave inside

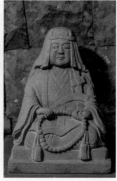

Waichi's sitting statue in the cave

◎ Bentenzai and Gemstone Cleansing Place

Within the shrine, close by the pond called Benten pond, there is a Benten statue created in 2014. There is a small washing place where you can cleanse your coins and precious stones for the grace of Benzaiten Goddess. Ejima Sugiyama Shrine grant precious stones for visitors called Mitamaishi in Japanese, they can be cleansed here to pray for long-lasting health and beauty, as the blessing of Benzaiten, as she has been a symbol of beauty (and other

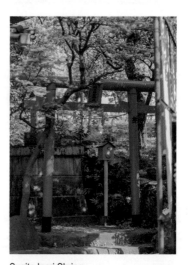

Sugita Inari Shrine

benefits) for many centuries. In Japanese, precious stones are also symbols of beauty, hence they are together in the shrine. Also, cleansing your own coins here benefits economic fortune, as Benzaiten is also a symbol of economic fortune.

◎ The Ruin of Sokumyou-an Hermitage

This hermitage was originally established to pray for Waichi's spirit by

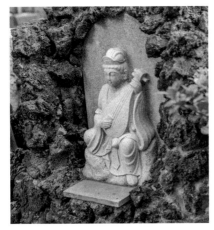

Benten statue near Benten pond

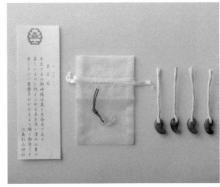

Mitamaishi (precious stone)

his apprentices after Waichi passed away. Later, the ruin was rebuilt in 1965, on the anniversary of Waichi's death.

◎ The Monument of Waichi Sugiyama

The monument was created in 1924 to commemorate the accomplishment of Waichi, as posthumous honors were conferred on him. This is the only monument in the world with all its writing in braille.

◎ Lifting Stone

The lifting stones are the large, heavy stones used for contests of strength and amusement, especially popular in the Edo era. In Tokyo Sumida-ku, there are 37 lifting stones from this time around, and this lifting stone is the heaviest among them, weighing 348.75kg (about 769lb).

◎ Mikoshiko: Stonehouse for Portable Shrine

The stonehouse stored all Mikoshi (portable shrine) in town. In 1929, using contributions from the shrines supporters, it was re-built with concrete to be sturdier and more protected. Then in 1945, during the biggest air raid of World War II, Benzaiten statue, hanging scrolls and biwa

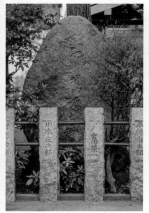 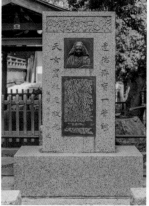 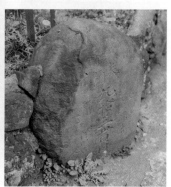

The Ruin of Sokumyou-an Hermitage   The Monument of Waichi Sugiyama   The "Lifting Stone"

musical instruments were brought here to protect them from fire. By this air raid, the main shrine was burned down, and the cave was partially destroyed, but this Mikoshiko survived. The ginkgo tree on the side of the stonehouse became carbonized by this big fire, but the root was not dead. The tree is still alive and fresh green leaves grow nowadays.

◎ Biwa instrument "Sazanami"

There is a previous biwa instrument stored in the shrine. Originally, the biwa was made by a famous biwa creator in Kyoto, and kept hidden in the castle of a high-ranking officer from 1789-1801. The feudal lord looked after it, then the highest-ranking blind officer received it from the lord, and gave it to one of his apprentices in 1862 as appreciation for his great contribution. It is said the biwa was historically held and sometimes played by high achieving blind officers.

In modern times, it was repaired in 2000 and 2016. When it was inspected in 2000, there was a record that it was repaired in 1823 and 1858. Biwa is known to record its repair timing inside of the main body.

Honjo "One Eye" mansion used to hold two big celebrations every year, following the tradition of Kyoto. During these occasions, biwa

instrument was played. This special biwa Sazanami was used for making beautiful music during such special occasions. The musical scenes are illustrated in some Japanese literature from that time.

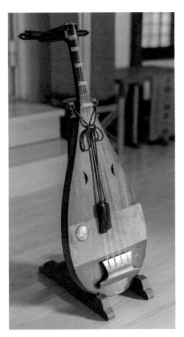

The historic biwa "Sazanami"

◎ Sugiyama Waichi Memorial Hall

There is Sugiyama Waichi Memorial Hall in the corner of the shrine. This hall was created in 2016 April to realize Waichi's lifetime passion of "acupuncture treatment education and study school." This is led by the Public Incorporated Foundation of Kengyo Sugiyama Kenshokai (Honoring Association) to commemorate Waichi's 400-year anniversary. The two-floor building has a multipurpose room on the first floor, and a material room to exhibit historical items on the second floor. There is an eastern medical clinic called "Sugiyama Acupuncture and Anma Clinic" inside as well. In the material room, there are historically important hanging scrolls such as Tunayoshi Shogunate's "Dai-Benzaiten" and "Rokkasen" plus many exhibitions related to Waichi Sugiyama and his work, acupuncture and anma history in Japan, including more than 400 literatures, 40 acupuncture tools and a small acupuncture point mannequin actually used during and after the Edo era. This second-floor material room was appointed by Sumida-ku, Tokyo as one of the collections of cultural items, literature and tools related to the history of the district.

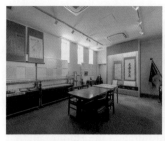

The Material Room inside

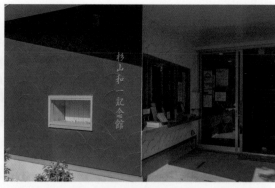

Sugiyama Waichi Memorial Hall (entrance)

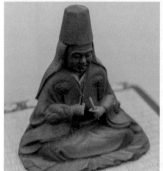

Waichi Sugiyama statue

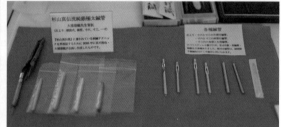

Pure silver extra large Shinkan and other Shinkan

The Spirits and Gods

◎ Ichikishimahime-no-mikoto – Benzaiten

Ejima Sugiyama shrine worshiped Benzaiten from Enoshima Island, but the deity is actually called Ichikishimahime-no-mikoto, she is the sea and water goddess appearing in Japanese mythology. She is one of the three well-known goddesses created by the oath between Amaterasu Omikami (Sun Goddess) and Susanoo-no-Mikoto (younger brother to Amaterasu). In the book called "the Chronicles of Japan," also called "Nihon-Shoki," she is the third goddess created in the world. In the book "Kojiki" (also called "Records of Ancient Matters") which is the oldest historical record of Japan, it states that she is the second goddess in the world. Amaterasu and Susanoo created eight gods, five male gods and three goddesses, and these three goddesses are called "Munakata Three Goddesses."

When syncretism of Shinto and Buddhism occurred, Ichikishimahime-no-mikoto was seen as the same as Benzaiten which came from China with the arrival of Buddhism. This syncretism was a phenomenon of merging two religions or symbols of religions, after recognition of similarities between the local religion and the newly arrived religion. This occurred between the Japanese local original religion Shinto and the Buddhism that arrived from China in 6th century. The syncretism at that time was more or less the Japanese old local religious ideas were merged with the new and popular one from China at that time. This phenomenon made Benzaiten and Ichikishimahimenomikoto into one symbol, and either of them to be seen both in shrines and temples.

Much later on, in 19th century the Japanese government in the Meiji era, aimed to bring modernity after the Edo era. They favored the Japanese original religion, and started prohibiting this merging practice. The government made a policy to make clear differentiations between shrines and temples. So many shrines who worshipped Benzaiten had to change it to either Ichikishimahimenomikoto or Munakata Three goddesses.

◎ Sarasvatī

Sarasvatī is known as the most beautiful goddess in Hinduism, and is known as the incarnation of the sacred river in Rigveda, a collection of ancient Indian hymns. She is widely known as a symbol of art, music, wisdom, learning and speech and ubiquitously seen in almost all nations in east Asia. Each country worships this goddess in many different forms. Originally, she was the goddess of water and good harvests, but later became more known for art and academia, and also became a symbol of warriors. Her drawings and statues have many different forms and shapes but most commonly she is illustrated as having four

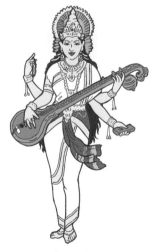

Sarasvatī

or eight arms. When she is drawn to have four arms, two arms hold the veda (Hindu bible) and rosary, and remaining arms hold a stringed instrument called veena/vena, which looks similar to biwa. When she has eight arms, often she is a symbol of warriors, so arms hold weapons such as bow, katana, short and long axes, halberd, iron ring and rope. When Sarasvatī went to China, she became a part of Buddhism in China and named as Benzaiten. Then eventually, arrived in Japan with Buddhism.

◎ Benzaiten

The oldest record addressing Benzaiten originating from Sarasvatī is "Dainichikyosho" which was written in 8th century China at the time of the Tang Dynasty. In the Buddhist scripture, Benzaiten was for wisdom, longevity and good fortune. Similar to Sarasvatī, Benzaiten is also known to be a warrior symbol, so often she was illustrated to have either four or eight arms and when she has eight arms, all of them were holding combat tools. So: Sarasvatī is Bentenzai and Bentenzai is Ichikishimahime-no-mikoto. People started calling Benzaiten and Ichikishimahime-no-mikoto interchangeably, and it was natural for them, as these two goddesses were both known to be very beautiful goddesses of water.

Benzaiten's form evolved uniquely in Japan. She came to have only two arms and holding biwa instrument. She is holding biwa as the original

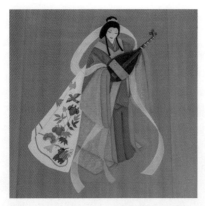
Benzaiten goddess merged with Japanese goddess

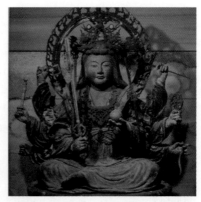
Benzaiten with eight arms

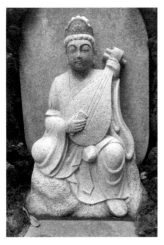
Benzaiten with veena (musical instrument)

Sarasvatī was holding the veena musical instrument. Also, by the Kamakura era in 13th century, Benzaiten was also merged with Ugajin, another god of fortune, and became worshipped as "Uga Benzaiten." This version has her head has a tiny Ugajin on top. As Ugajin has snakes and dragons on his body, when merged with Benzaiten, the snakes and dragons became the messengers for the Benzaiten. These creatures were not seen elsewhere in east Asia, only in Japan. Further, in Japan, Benzaiten is also called "Benten" as a short name, and worshipped as a treasure goddess. According to the old literature, the magic spell of Benzaiten brought desirable treasures. This literature created the belief of Benzaiten. In a shrine called "Zeni-arai Benzaiten Ugajinja" in Kamakura city, Kanagawa prefecture, it is believed to bring a lot of economic fortune by cleansing coins in the natural spring water stream in the cave inside the shrine precincts. In modern times, Benzaiten became one of the "Seven Gods of Good Fortune" members (well known as "Shichi-Fukujin" in Japan) and worshipped to bring luck and fortune. As Benten became popular, the shrines who worship Benzaiten started calling themselves as "Benten Shrine." As it enshrines Benzaiten, Ejima Sugiyama shrine was also called "Honjo One Eye Benten Shrine."

As both Sarasvatī-Benzaiten and Ichikishimahime-no-mikoto are goddesses of water, it is common that Benzaiten shrines were built nearby water - sea, rivers and lakes, many built on islands and shores. As Benzaiten became more popular and widely worshipped, more Benzaiten shrines were created. In such shrines, it is considered a lucky day of Benzaiten is know as the "snake day" which is the sixth sign of Chinese zodiac, and "double snake day" is even better, bringing lots of luck. The double snake day comes once in sixty days.

◎ Ugajin

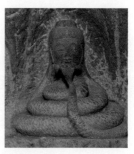

Ugashin statue

In Ejima Sugiyama shrine, there is a Ugajin god worshipped in the cave in the shrine precincts. Ugajin is a well-known god in Japan, often depicted with a body of snake loafing around, or the body of dragon, and head can be a man or woman. Where the name "Uga" came from is not clear, but it has been considered to be worshipped for good grain and fortune, and when it was adapted by Tendai Buddhism, it was fused to Benzaiten. As addressed above, Ugajin-Benzaiten is called as "Uga-Benzaiten" and depicted as Benzaiten with small Ugajin on top of her head. The Ejima shrine in Enoshima Island, which was deeply worshipped by Waichi Sugiyama, had a "Uga-Benzaiten." Hence, it is believed appropriate to have Ugajin in Ejima Sugiyama shrine as well.

Characteristics of Ejima Sugiyama Shrine

◎ Ichikishimahime-no-mikoto and Waichi Sugiyama

Ejima Sugiyama shrine's uniqueness comes from what it enshrined - Ichikishimahime-no-mikoto, or Benzaiten and Sarasvatī are all known as beautiful water goddesses, and were worshipped for good fortune, wisdom and longevity. On the other hand, Waichi Sugiyama is the spirit of Japanese traditional medicine. He was known for his impeccable achievement healing the disease of Tsunayoshi Tokugawa, the fifth Shogun, and worked as a personal doctor for him. Plus, he lived till 85, an exceptionally long life at that time. Ejima Sugiyama shrine is the only one in the world to worship them together, so the benefit of it are numerous, relating to health, beauty and longevity, as well as good fortune and wisdom.

◎ Precious Stones and Special Cleansing Place

Further, another unique aspect of Ejima Sugiyama shrine is to offer Mitamaishi (precious stones) as shrine's grants for visitors and there is a

103

small cleansing place for them. Visitors can cleanse and pray for long-lasting youth, health and beauty, as the blessing of Bentenzai God who has been a symbol of beauty since ancient time and Waichi who was a symbol of health and longevity.

As the shrine enshrines Benzaiten and Waichi Sugiyama together, Ejima Sugiyama shrine became

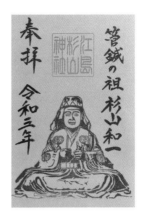

Goshuin (a stamp) from Ejima Sugiyama Shrine

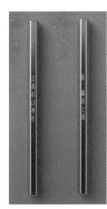

Shinkan-shaped lucky charms

known as a "power spot" for health, beauty and longevity. Modern Japan realizes the life span of 100 years as a norm, and the society is changing to embrace longer-life. Japanese people's wishes of health and beauty is getting ever higher. Many visitors to benefit enshrined deities from Bentenzai and Waichi Sugiyama.

◎ Improve Acupuncture Treatment Skill, Achieve Shinkyu, Anma Study and Practice, and Passing National Board Exams

Also, as Wachi Sugiyama was worshipped as the spirit of Japanese Shinkyu, many professional acupuncturists and students of eastern medicine visit the shrine to pray for advancing acupuncture skill, successful completion of Shinkyu education and also pray for passing the national board exam.

On the second floor of shrine, there is a material room with many exceptional historical writings, references and tools for Japanese Shinkyu being exhibited. For people who practice acupuncture or moxibustion, or enjoy Shinkyu, Ejima Sugiyama shrine and Sugiyama Waichi Memorial Hall are 'must-see' places.

Chapter 8

The Birthplace of Kanshin Method

Enoshima Shrine and the Original Cave

Enoshima Shrine where Waichi Sugiyama fasted and prayed for inspiration from the god is located in Fujisawa City, Kanagawa prefecture. It is said that the Shrine was started from the caves, which were built by the imperial command coming from the Emperor Kinmei (AC 510-571). There are two caves that were originally created by the erosion from the sea. The current sizes are rather small at 152m and 56m each, respectively. Until Edo period, Benzaiten (the gods of multiple benefits, explained in the previous chapter) were enshrined here, and thus the Shrine was nicknamed as "Enoshima Benten" or "Enoshima Myojin" and attracted utmost respect as the top spiritual shrine of the Kanto region. Later, as the Meiji period government's policy changed to separate Japanese local gods from Buddhism, it became a Shrine to present three gods simultaneously. The sanctuary was divided into three sites: the "Hetsu-miya" shrine to present the Japanese local god, and "middle" shrine and "rear" shrines to

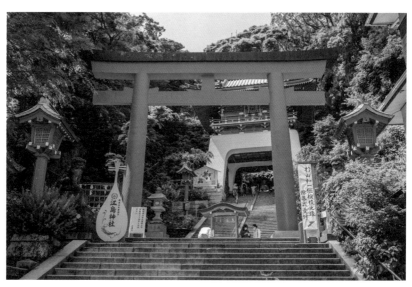

Tori-I (front guard frame) at Enoshima Shrine (Kanagawa, Japan)

Waichi Sugiyama sitting statue

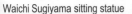

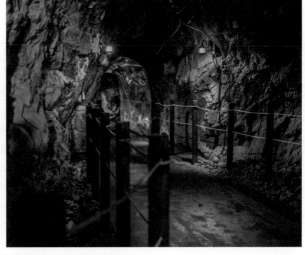

Inside of the original cave

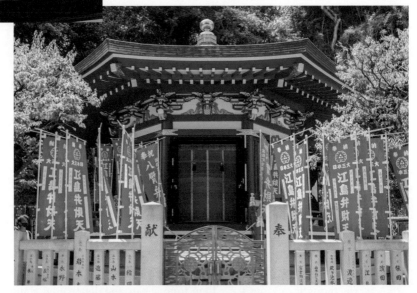

Hou-An-Den (enshrine the gods)

present different gods. The "rear" shrine is the closest to the original caves, hence it was called the central shrine. Hetsu-miya is located at the lowest level within the Shrine so called as "bottom" shrine.

In these three sites, each site used to have a lodging facility to support

the "Okomori" training. This is a Buddhist worship discipline praying for the god's inspiration while fasting for days. In this place, it is said famous Japanese Buddhist teachers, such as Saint Kobo and Nichiren, stayed and prayed in this Shrine. Waichi stayed in the bottom shrine for 21 days without foods, and praying in the cave to seek great god's oracle.

After the Meiji era, with the modernization and westernization of Japan, the lodging facility became a regular Ryokan (Japanese style hotel, Bed and Breakfast) not a part of any religion. One of these hotel accommodations became famous, called "Kinkiro Enoshima" hotel, which was known for its luxurious and famous seaside view, but is now gone. Currently, there are several important statues stored in a temple called Hou-An-Den in the premises, including Happi Benzaiten, Myo-on Benzaiten and Waichi Sugiyama's wooden sitting statue.

The Statues of Waichi Sugiyama

2020 was the 410-year anniversary of the birth of Waichi Sugiyama. Fujisawa City Acupuncture and Massage Therapist Association, a local professional association that has a deep connection with Waichi, planned to build a statue of him within the Ejima Shrine. In June 2019, when a board member visited Ejima Shrine to talk about their plan, the chief priest said that they already have a statue of Waichi. When the board member saw the statue, he found a wooden sitting statue of Waichi, around 50cm height. It is the only statue ordered by Waichi when he was alive.

The statue was kept in the storage room behind the Shrine, but no one really knew where came from or how long it was kept there. Among the people who knew the fact that Waichi made this statue when he was alive, it was thought missing for a long time. Then, the discovered statue had a mark stating "Mister Sugiyama, May 18th in 1685" in a good condition. Enoshima Shrine asked Mr. Kazuo Usui, a local well-known historian working at a history museum for an appraisal. They received the authentic answer: the statue was created by Waichi's order, and can be "a first-class Buddhist statue, and can even be a national treasure." Currently, it is kept

at the Shrine after being polished into perfect shape again.

On the other hand, the Waichi's statue to commemorate the 410-year anniversary was successfully built and settled at the side of "the lucky stone" within the shrine. It was unveiled to the public on September 4th in 2020 with the ceremony of the new statue. It is said that the "lucky stone" was the stone Waichi tripped over at the end of his fasting worship when he was inspired by the idea of creating acupuncture guide tubes. After tripping over this stone, Waichi's life was turned around to be successful. So it is believed this stone brought success.

Both the original wooden statue and new statue created recently are displayed together side by side at the Enoshima Shrine.

Reference:
Kanagawa and Tokyo Tama-region local information magazine
Town News Fujisawa City
Issued:
February 28, 2020
September 11, 2020

*I*t has been a wonderful journey to work with Kitagawa sensei to publish the first bilingual book ever to share the essence of Japanese Shinkyu. Every time I received a Japanese manuscript, I learned a lot and deepened my appreciation of the "father of Japanese acupuncture," Waichi Sugiyama's work. He innovated and evolved the Japanese Shinkyu to become what it is today: a gentle yet powerful healing modality.

*A*s a Japanese acupuncturist overseas, I always tell my patients that "we (Japanese) use very thin needles to make you feel more comfortable. Yet the effect is magnificent." With Japanese style, I believe acupuncture can be kind and efficient. In fact, in the U.S, most people who do not want to try acupuncture are afraid of needle insertion pain. I wish all of them can try Japanese Shinkyu and receive the comfortable, effective treatment. This is all possible thanks to the fact that Waichi changed the map of acupuncture forever by creating Shinkan (guide tube) in the seventeenth century.

*I*am honored to be a part of this book. I cannot thank enough Kitagawa sensei to trust me to do this massive work. I thank all the people who are involved to make this beautiful bilingual book come true. I also thank my husband, Martin, who supported me. I hope this book encourages practitioners to talk more about Japanese Shinkyu and to let it be known globally. We can also let the world know that Shinkan – guide tube was actually born and raised in Japan. I sincerely wish to increase the awareness of Japanese Shinkyu at the global level, as the world needs more of the Japanese Shinkyu.

From my clinic in Paris 12eme,
Midori McGivern
D.Ac., L.Ac, M.S, M.P.S.

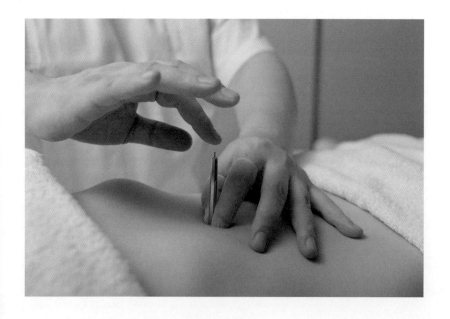